THE ENABLING ENVIRONMENT FOR EPIDEMIC AND PANDEMIC RISK FINANCING IN PAKISTAN

COUNTRY DIAGNOSTICS ASSESSMENT

DECEMBER 2024

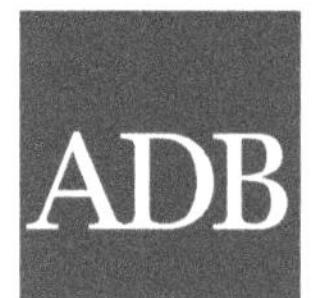

ASIAN DEVELOPMENT BANK

Contents

Tables, Figures, and Boxes

Acknowledgments

This report was prepared under the Technical Assistance-6561 REG: Strengthening the Enabling Environment for Disaster Risk Financing (Phase 2). The Technical Assistance was executed by the Asian Development Bank (ADB) in collaboration with the Government of Pakistan.

Charlotte Benson, principal disaster risk management specialist, Climate Change and Disaster Risk Management Division, Climate Change and Sustainable Development Department, ADB; and Arup Chatterjee, principal financial sector specialist, Finance Sector Office, Sectors Group, ADB, provided direction and technical advice for this report.

The report benefited significantly from discussions with and comments from Yong Ye, Country Director, ADB Pakistan Resident Mission (PRM), Central and West Asia Department (CWRD); Mian Shafi, Senior Project Officer, (PRM), CWRD; Salman Mian, Senior Project Officer, (PRM), CWRD; Asif Turangzai, Project Officer, (PRM), CWRD; Hiddo Huitzing, Senior Health Specialist, Human and Social Development Division, CWRD; and Andrew McCartney, Senior Financial Sector Economist, Public Management, Financial Sector, and Trade Division, CWRD.

The report was produced by a team of ADB consultants comprising international consultants Rodolfo Wehrhahn (team leader, insurance and capital market regulatory specialist), Christian Pfleiderer (health insurance specialist), Sheraz Ahmad Khan (national consultant, insurance industry specialist), and ADB consultant Maria Cristina Pascual (project coordinator).

The report benefited extensively from interaction with organizations to whom the team would like to express great appreciation for representatives for their time and candidness.

Government Agencies
Ministry of Finance (Department of Budget and Accounts)
Ministry of National Health Services Regulations and Coordination
Ministry of Planning and Development (Planning Commission of Pakistan)
Ministry of Economic Affairs
National Disaster Management Authority
National Disaster Reduction Management Fund
Small and Medium Enterprise Development Authority
Security and Exchange Commission of Pakistan
Benazir Income Support Programme
Sehat Sahulat Program (Khyber Pakhtunkhwa and Federal)
Punjab Provincial Government (Department of Health)

Public Limited Companies and State-Owned Enterprises
State Life Insurance Corporation

Private Sector
Jubilee Insurance
Pak-Qatar Family Takaful
Pakistan Microfinance Network

Development Partners
Deutsche Gesellschaft für Internationale Zusammenarbeit (GIZ)
KfW
World Health Organization, Pakistan
United Nations International Children's Emergency Fund, Pakistan

Abbreviations

ADB	–	Asian Development Bank
BISP	–	Benazir Income Support Programme
COVID-19	–	coronavirus disease
DRF	–	disaster risk financing
GDP	–	gross domestic product
IRCM	–	insurance, reinsurance, and capital market
OECD	–	Organisation for Economic Co-operation and Development
SECP	–	Securities and Exchange Commission of Pakistan
SLIC	–	State Life Insurance Corporation
SSP	–	Sehat Sahulat Program
TA	–	Technical Assistance
WHO	–	World Health Organization

Currency Equivalent

Currency Unit	=	Pakistan rupee (PRs)
PRs1.00	=	$0.0035467281
$1.00	=	PRs281.95

Executive Summary

The coronavirus disease pandemic tested Pakistan's financing capacity resulting in a long-lasting and severe impact on the economy, including medical costs, lower productivity and unemployment during lockdowns, and trade and supply chain interruptions. As such, governments and businesses need to prepare financially for pandemics and epidemics in ways similar to that for extreme weather or geophysical events.

This country diagnostic assesses Pakistan's current disaster risk financing landscape and enabling environment for the efficient and effective use of existing epidemic and pandemic financing instruments and the introduction of new ones to enhance financial resilience. The assessment covers both risk retention and risk transfer instruments. It completes an earlier assessment of the enabling environment for disasters triggered by natural hazards in Pakistan (ADB 2019).

The assessment of the enabling environment for the effective use of risk retention instruments is based on a joint Asian Development Bank and World Bank (2017) questionnaire. This questionnaire has been adjusted to include epidemic and pandemic risk financing.

The assessment of the enabling environment for the effective use of risk transfer instruments to the insurance, reinsurance, and capital markets is based on a modified version of the "W&W Development Framework." It focuses on six areas of relevance for the development of epidemic and pandemic insurance, reinsurance, and capital market solutions: (1) economic conditions and other support functions; (2) government policy; (3) social protection policy; (4) unlicensed competition; (5) credibility of insurance, reinsurance, and capital markets providers; and (6) product appeal.

A risk layered structure is proposed to stimulate, develop, and implement financially sustainable and scalable disaster risk financing strategies and solutions.

Recommendations to enhance the enabling environment for epidemic and pandemic risk financing have been drawn from the assessment. The list of recommendations is presented below.

Key Recommendations to Strengthen the Enabling Environment for Epidemic and Pandemic Risk Financing

Recommendations	Timing and References
The implementation of the key recommendations provided by the external evaluation for International Health Regulations (IHR) and Global Health Security Agenda core capacities were interrupted by the coronavirus disease (COVID-19) outbreak. ***Continue progress toward full implementation of the key recommendations provided by the external evaluation for IHR and Global Health Security Agenda core capacities.***	Immediate. Para. 51
At the onset of the pandemic, Pakistan suffered from a deficiency of human health resources, deficiencies in the routine health system data, and limited availability of public health laboratories. ***Provide targeted investments in the health system to reduce epidemic and pandemic risk.***	Near term. Para. 53
The existing data systems are fragmented and not integrated and the data system for COVID-19 case reporting had to be set up ad hoc during the pandemic. ***Work toward integrated and effective health data and reporting systems, integrating the private providers.***	Near term. Para. 54
The COVID-19 pandemic data has yet to be completed and used for the development of epidemic and pandemic risk models. ***Use available COVID-19 data once the National Disaster Management Agency has completed collection, for the development of sophisticated pandemic and epidemic risk models.***	Near term. Para. 55
A federal coordination center for pandemic response was established on an ad-hoc basis. The 2016 World Health Organization evaluation recommended the establishment of such a body within the Ministry of National Health Services Regulations and Coordination. ***Put in place legislation, protocols, funding sources, etc., to facilitate rapid mobilization of coordination centers in response to major disasters.***	Immediate. Para. 37
While the provincial governments are responsible for health care, their insufficient contingent funds delayed containment of the pandemic. ***Review the current allocation of contingent funds for disasters, pandemics/epidemics at provincial level.***	Near term. Para. 38
The Auditor General of Pakistan said government departments lacked preparedness to respond to the pandemics and financial controls were weak. ***Address any areas that require additional explanation and guidance on the exemption clauses to the Public Procurement Regulatory Authority rule.***	Near term. Para. 39

continued on next page

Table   *continued*

Recommendations	Timing and References
Neither the federal nor the KP Sehat Sahulat Program (SSP) have funds allocated for responding to pandemics/epidemics. *Include coverage for pandemics/epidemics in the SSP package and price actuarially for pandemic/epidemic cover when purchasing insurance for the SSP. Implement the federal SSP planned reserve fund to finance any unforeseen health care emergency or catastrophe and revise the benefits package to include pandemics/epidemics.*	Near term. Para. 75
Health care needs relating to the COVID-19 pandemic were financed completely by the government, with no risk transfer instruments supporting the budget. *Explore possible acquisition of pandemic and epidemic risk transfer instruments that provide funds at the points of need for the federal government to enhance the risk layered approach to epidemics/pandemics financing if economically viable.*	Immediate. Para. 79
Forward-looking financial supervision instruments in the form of stress testing of events such as long-lasting pandemics are not in place. *Require the insurance sector to develop and carry out stress testing under epidemic and pandemic scenarios like the COVID-19 pandemic (for the SSP).*	Near term, Para. 86
The benefits remains fully funded by the government, with limited risk transfer to the insurance sector. *Consider transferring part of the health risk, including pandemic and epidemic, to additional insurers in the SSPs, with eventual support from reinsurance.*	Near term, Para. 87
All health claims-related data from the SSP is only available to the government and State Life Insurance Corporation, hindering an efficient pricing of supplementary health insurance products by the whole insurance sector. *Make all health claims-related data from the SSP available to the insurance sector while complying with privacy regulations.*	Near term. Para. 89
Significant pandemic-related business revenue losses have remained uninsured. *Consider multiyear business interruption insurance that includes epidemics/pandemics from specialized insurers for government to support businesses.*	Immediate. Para. 92
The importance of the Ehsaas is indisputable but availability of funds was challenging due to the financial stress created by the COVID-19 and the competing needs for government funding. *Acquire a risk transfer instrument for the Ehsaas programs that provides funds in the event of a pandemic or major epidemic.*	Near term. Para. 101

KP = Khyber Pakhtunkhwa.
Note: "Immediate" is within 1 year. "Near term" is 1 to 3 years.
Source: Asian Development Bank.

Introduction

1.1 Background

1.   The **Asian Development Bank (ADB) conducted a country diagnostic of the enabling environment for disaster risk financing (DRF) for Pakistan in 2019 (ADB 2019).** The report covered natural hazards affecting the country, including earthquakes, cyclones, floods, and droughts. The report provided a series of recommendations, including 14 key recommendations for Strengthening of the Enabling Environment for Disaster Risk Financing that the government considered and several of which that have or are to be implemented.

2.   **This report also provides supplementary analysis extending the scope of the initial diagnostic to cover epidemics and pandemics.** The severity and long duration of the coronavirus disease (COVID-19) pandemic tested the financial resilience of countries across the globe. Its severe economic impact created unprecedented financing challenges in addressing health needs, providing livelihoods and business relief support, and maintaining economic stability. This situation of financial stress for the country on top of the financial needs caused by disasters due to natural hazards has motivated ADB to include in its assessment of the enabling environment for disaster risk financing the epidemics and pandemics to the natural hazards already covered.

3.   **The different nature of the financial impact of disasters triggered by natural hazards and those caused by long-lasting epidemics and pandemics requires differing financial instruments and enabling measures.** Figure 1 illustrates the different timeline and areas of loss impacted by disasters and epidemics and pandemics.

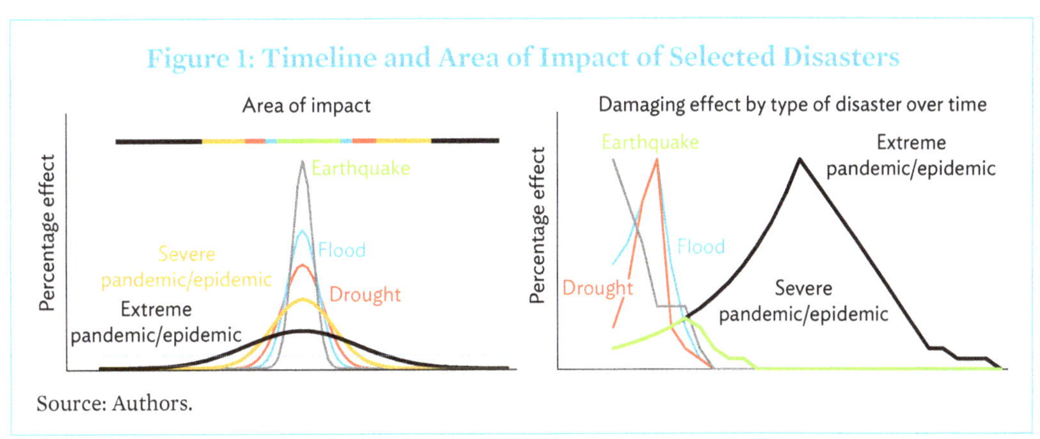

Source: Authors.

4.   **Enhanced financial preparedness for disasters is an ADB priority.** The technical assistance (TA) project, *Strengthening the Enabling Environment for Disaster Risk Financing (Phase 2)*, under which this report is prepared, is consistent with ADB's 2021 Disaster and Emergency Assistance Policy, which explicitly supports enhanced financing arrangements for disasters, epidemics, and pandemics (ADB 2021). It is also consistent with the Financial Sector Directional Guide under development, which calls for building capabilities in emerging and innovative finance areas such DRF.[1]

5.   **ADB's holistic approach to DRF is reflected in this TA.** ADB strongly advocates an integrated approach to disaster and emergency risk management to strengthen resilience through risk reduction and enhanced management of residual risk. ADB seeks to enhance financial preparedness for disasters, pandemics, and epidemics as part of broader efforts to strengthen resilience to these events. This is done in close coordination with governments, global and regional DRF initiatives,[2] standard-setting bodies (the International Association of Insurance Supervisors, and the International Organization of Securities Commissions), the Basel Committee on Banking Supervision, the Islamic Financial Services Board, the Financial Stability Institute, and the insurance industry. Risk reduction efforts should be the first consideration in addressing disaster, pandemic, and epidemic risk, tackling the root causes of the issue. DRF solutions should also conform with international financial standards and be designed around the context of broader disaster, pandemic and epidemic resilience; financial stability; and financial inclusion, incorporating incentives for risk reduction. This approach should lead to the development and implementation of financially sustainable, scalable DRF strategies and solutions. ADB applies a risk-layered approach to support the appropriate selection of disaster, pandemic, and epidemic risk management options, including DRF instruments.

6.   **This country diagnostic assessment identifies areas of improvement to promote an enhanced enabling environment for the financial risk management of pandemics and epidemics.** Notwithstanding the importance of risk financing instruments, these can only be fully effective under certain conditions that are often neglected. Assessing and identifying barriers to be removed to create an enabling environment for increased uptake of these instruments is critical. This country diagnostic is intended to facilitate the development and implementation of appropriate instruments for different layers of risk. It identifies areas of improvement to enhance the enabling environment for public sector DRF solutions as well as for insurance, reinsurance, and capital market (IRCM) solutions.

7.   **Recommendations based on the assessment are comprehensively presented in the corresponding sections.** The recommended activities and measures to enhance the enabling environment for key public sector DRF instruments, as well as IRCM solutions, are presented at the end of the relevant section. A summary of the main recommendations are listed in the executive summary.

---

[1]   The term "disaster risk financing" is used in this report to include risk financing for pandemics and epidemics as well as disasters triggered by natural hazards.

[2]   These include the InsuResilience Global Partnership; Vulnerable Twenty (V20) Group; the Insurance Development Forum; the Disaster Risk Financing and Insurance Program of the World Bank, Market Global Practice and Global Facility for Disaster Reduction and Recovery; the Pacific Disaster Risk Financing and Insurance Program; and the Asia-Pacific Economic Cooperation and the Organisation for Economic Co-operation and Development Promoting the G20/OECD Methodological Framework for Disaster Risk Assessment and Risk Financing.

1.2   Economic Impact of a Severe Pandemic: Coronavirus Disease

8.   **The COVID-19 pandemic's impact was twofold:** it directly impacted health systems and health parameters and affected economies, livelihoods, and poverty through the reactions of populations and governments, and the measures taken to curb its spread; and the impact on livelihoods and poverty rates.

9.   Worldwide, over 590 million people were reported to have been infected and more than 6.4 million deaths recorded as of mid-2022.[3] However, World Health Organization (WHO) estimates point to more than 50% higher figures.[4] Incidence and mortality figures also varied widely across countries due to differing population structures and health system performance.

10.   **Countries launched their individual programs for testing and surveillance, protective equipment for health workers, and scaling up of treatment facilities.** These expenses, however, were at least partly compensated by the underutilization of the health systems for all other services due to lockdowns and people avoiding going to health facilities. This is mirrored in estimations of health care spending worldwide (Figure 2).

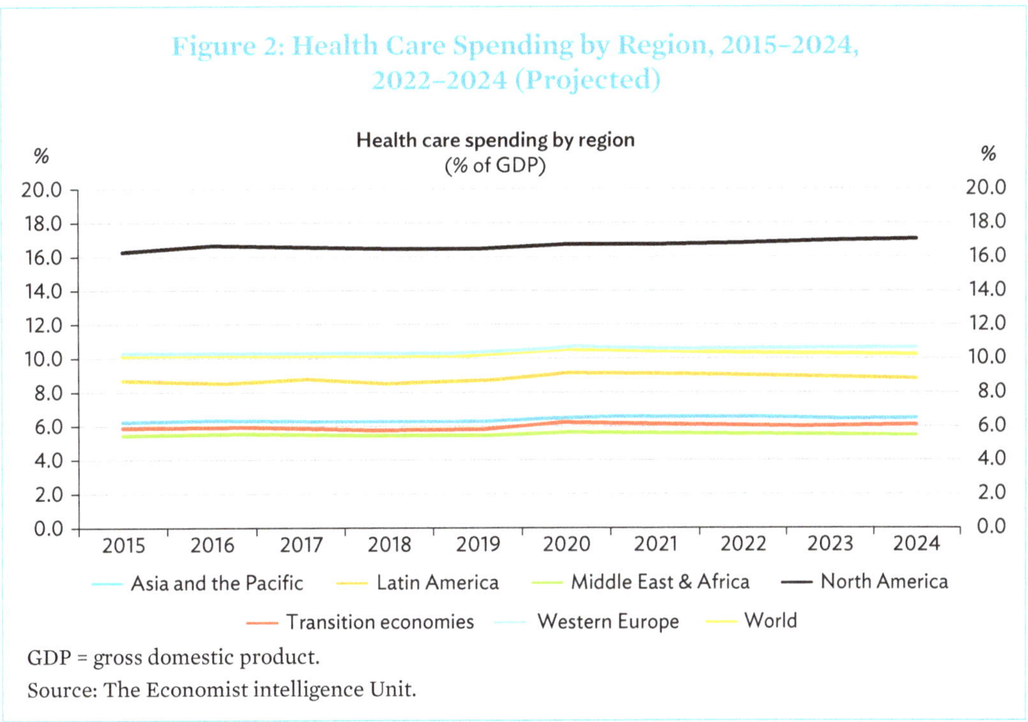

Figure 2: Health Care Spending by Region, 2015–2024, 2022–2024 (Projected)

GDP = gross domestic product.

Source: The Economist intelligence Unit.

11.   **The latest WHO report on global health expenditure shows a similar, albeit preliminary picture (WHO 2021), as for most of the countries, especially low- and middle-income brackets, no data is available yet.** Governments of the sample countries covered by

---

[3]   Worldometer. COVID-19 Live Statistics. https://www.worldometers.info/coronavirus/ (accessed 15 August 2022).

[4]   WHO. 2021. The True Death Toll of COVID-19: Estimating Global Excess Mortality. https://www.who.int/data/stories/the-true-death-toll-of-covid-19-estimating-global-excess-mortality.

the report increased their health expenditures by 8% on average, but with wide variation. The share of government health expenditure in total government expenditures, however, mostly decreased, as increases in health expenditure were surpassed by budget allocations to address the economic consequences of the pandemic and social protection. Private expenses in general mostly decreased, mirroring reduced health care-seeking behavior other than COVID-19-related utilization. However, in COVID-19 affected households, expenses increased, adding impoverishment to the pandemic effects.

12.   **Pandemic impact on the global economy was the most severe shock since the Second World War.** Lockdowns slashed economic activity and consumption and disrupted global supply chains. Gross domestic product (GDP) in high-income countries was hit harder than in low-income countries, the latter because of their more localized economic systems (Figure 3). Socioeconomically, however, the impact was worse for low- and middle-income countries, with their enterprises and employment much less able to cope and social protection systems far less developed. World Bank (2021) estimated that people living in poverty has increased by almost 100 million due to the global economic crisis (Figure 4).

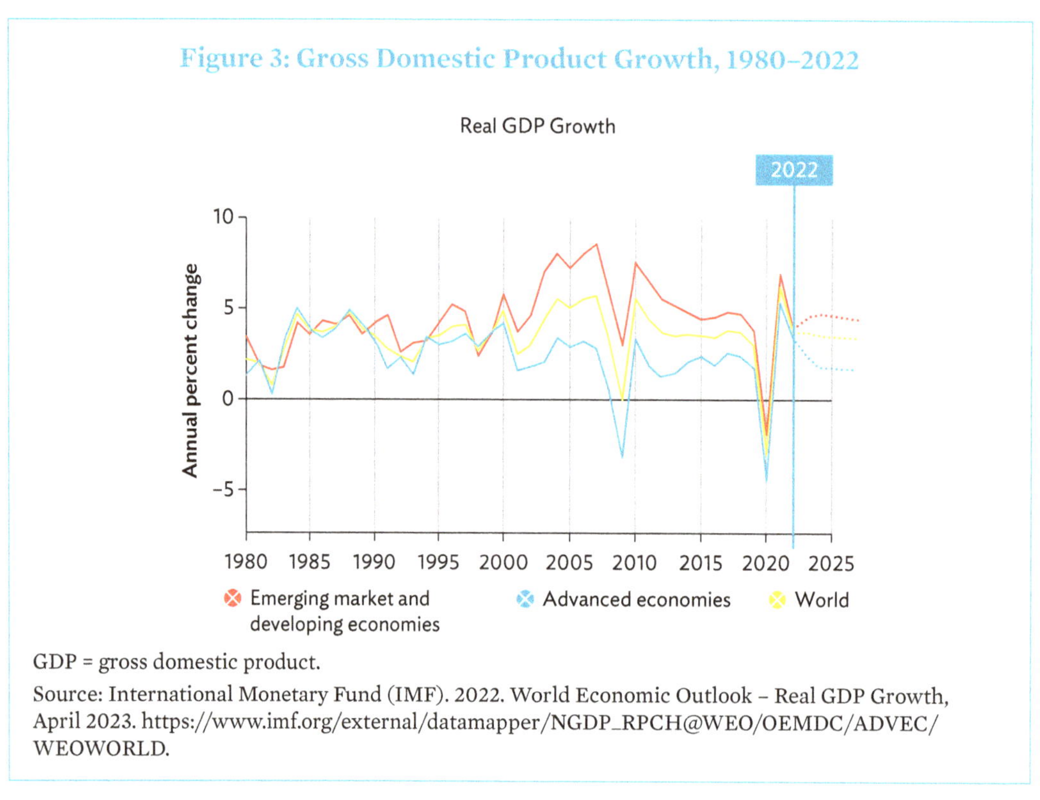

GDP = gross domestic product.

Source: International Monetary Fund (IMF). 2022. World Economic Outlook – Real GDP Growth, April 2023. https://www.imf.org/external/datamapper/NGDP_RPCH@WEO/OEMDC/ADVEC/WEOWORLD.

13.   Countries need to strengthen their financial resilience to pandemics and epidemics, and the appropriate instruments for this purpose will depend on a range of factors. The most appropriate bundle of instruments depends on the scale of resources required at each layer of loss relative to the scale of resources each instrument can facilitate access to (Figure 5); the speed with which funds are required relative to the disbursement speed of each instrument; the marginal cost of each instrument; individual country circumstances, including prevailing macroeconomic circumstances; the scale of potential events relative to GDP; government economic, fiscal, and monetary goals and objectives; access to international finance markets; and the market-based cost of borrowing (ADB 2013).

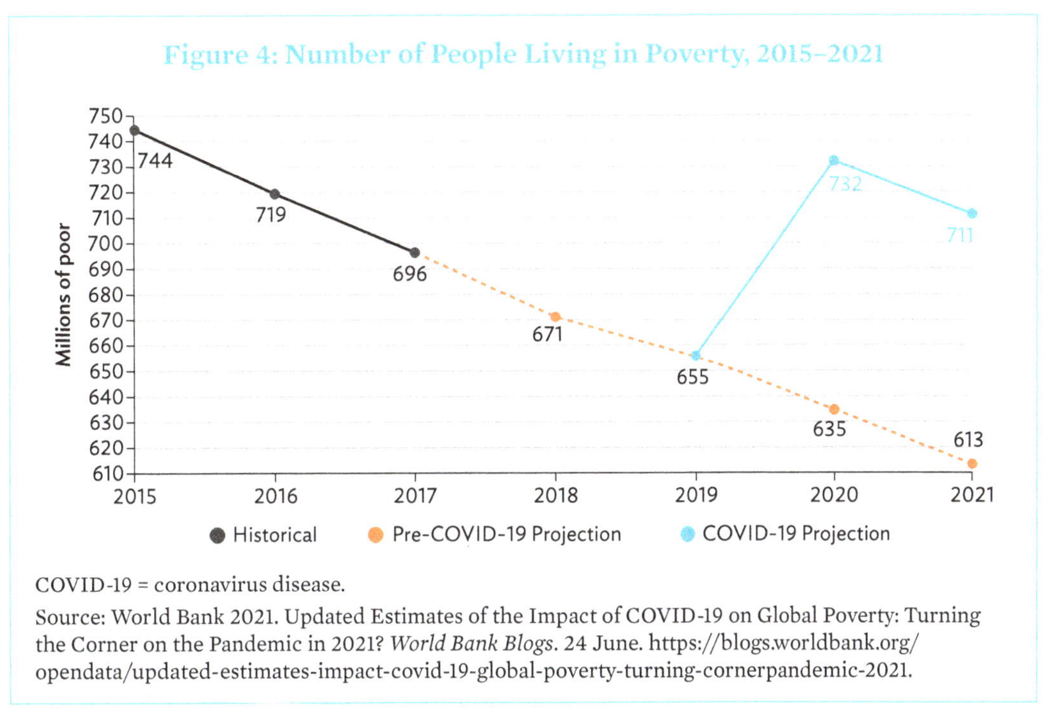

Figure 4: Number of People Living in Poverty, 2015–2021

COVID-19 = coronavirus disease.
Source: World Bank 2021. Updated Estimates of the Impact of COVID-19 on Global Poverty: Turning the Corner on the Pandemic in 2021? *World Bank Blogs*. 24 June. https://blogs.worldbank.org/opendata/updated-estimates-impact-covid-19-global-poverty-turning-cornerpandemic-2021.

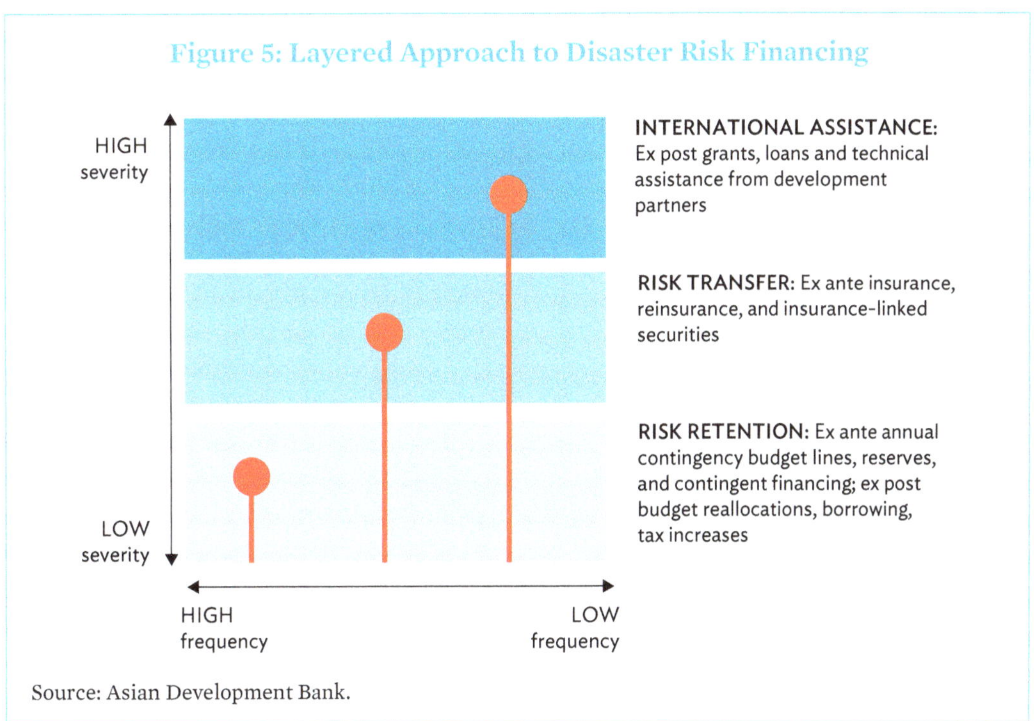

Figure 5: Layered Approach to Disaster Risk Financing

Source: Asian Development Bank.

For example, if probable maximum losses from extreme events are low relative to GDP, then a country is better able to retain risk. A country with low indebtedness can rely more on post-event borrowing than one with a higher level. The effectiveness of risk transfer instruments also depends crucially on the availability of well-developed and sound domestic insurance and capital market sectors. Among other issues, the cultural and religious dimensions are important, while it should be noted that government policy could potentially crowd in or out the private insurance sector.

1.3 Country Diagnostics Methodology

1.3.1 Diagnostic Tool

14.   This country diagnostics has been undertaken by applying a similar diagnostics tool to the one used in the assessment of Pakistan under Phase 1 of this TA project. The tool has been enhanced to assess the enabling environment for pandemic and epidemic risk financing instruments. The diagnostics tool covers both sovereign and nonsovereign risk financing instruments and generates an overview of current risk financing policies and mechanisms. It identifies enabling conditions for effective use of well-established risk financing instruments, the introduction of new instruments and related barriers and gaps; sets policy priorities for implementing reforms and introducing new instruments; and provides the basis for new or deeper engagement on DRF by governments, regulators, and development partners as part of broader epidemic and pandemic risk management and public financial management dialogue.

15.   The tool includes two structured questionnaires. The first questionnaire helps with the assessment of the framework used by the government to finance epidemics and pandemics within its budget, i.e., when risk is retained. The second questionnaire provides insights into risk transfer instruments. The two questionnaires are critical for evaluating the existing enabling environment for both risk retention and risk transfer instruments.

16.   The assessment of the enabling environment for the effective use of risk retention instruments is based on a joint ADB and World Bank (2017) questionnaire. This questionnaire has been adjusted to include epidemic and pandemic risk financing (Box 1).

17.   The assessment of the enabling environment for the effective use of risk transfer instruments is based on a modified version of the "W&W Development Framework."[5] This framework was refined to provide a methodology for assessing the pandemic and epidemic risk financing landscape and its enabling environment. It focuses on six areas relevant for the development of epidemic and pandemic IRCM solutions, as follows:

- *Economic conditions* and other support functions like the disposable budget for health insurance, covering pandemics and epidemics, the level of government indebtedness as well as data availability, health facilities, doctors, vaccines, and pandemic/epidemics research institutes; and other relevant professionals, e.g., actuaries, adjusters, accountants etc. necessary for the well-functioning of the providers of IRCM.
- *Government policy on the development of risk transfer instruments,* including the introduction of mandatory insurance protection, risk-pooling structures and insurance-linked securities,[6] pertinent regulations, and the creation of a level playing field for IRCM activities.

---

[5] The W&W Development Framework has been used on several occasions by Rodolfo Wehrhahn, one of the assessors, to determine barriers to an enabling environment in work done for ADB, the International Monetary Fund, and the World Bank. The relevant areas for an enabling environment as determined in this framework are based on Wehrhahn (2010).

[6] Insurance-linked securities bonds, including catastrophe bonds and other risk-linked securitization, represent assets whose value is largely driven by the occurrence of events not correlated to the financial markets, allowing for a high degree of diversification. With an insurance-linked securities bond, the investor is exposed to a well-defined catastrophic or insurable event in addition to the credit risk of the issuer. For this additional exposure, investors are compensated with higher coupons, but if no covered event occurs during the risk period, the bonds are redeemed at 100% of face value. When a covered event meets the thresholds in the risk transfer contract, investors stand to lose coupon payments and/or a percentage of the principal. The redemption price of the bonds is reduced accordingly. ADB (forthcoming) provides details.

Box 1: Examining the Full Sovereign Disaster Risk Financing Landscape

The enhanced and adapted Asian Development Bank–World Bank disaster risk financing diagnostic assesses sovereign financial protection against disasters. It includes questions on risk transfer sovereign arrangements but strongly focuses on risk retention mechanisms. The adapted version to address pandemics and epidemics covers the following issues:

1. Assessment of fiscal shocks associated with epidemics and pandemics
   - Contingent liability of the government
   - Fiscal risk assessment of epidemic and pandemic shocks
   - Public disclosure of fiscal exposure to epidemics and pandemics

2. *Ex-ante* risk financing instruments that can be used to finance the losses due to an epidemic or a pandemic
   - Annual contingency budget
   - Dedicated budget lines for risk reduction
   - Dedicated reserve funds
   - Line agency funding
   - Contingent credit and grant arrangements

3. *Ex post* risk financing instruments
   - Post-event budget reallocations
   - External assistance
   - Tax increments
   - Government borrowing

Source: Adapted from ADB and World Bank. 2017. *Assessing Financial Protection Against Disasters: A Guidance Note on Conducting a Disaster Risk Finance Diagnostic.*

- *Credibility of the private sector offering risk transfer* solutions covering issues such as the regulatory environment; the solvency of risk carriers; the reputation of insurance and capital markets, as well as the professionalism of distribution channels, loss adjusters, and brokers; and the availability of infrastructure (e.g., stock exchanges, payment systems, etc.).
- *Epidemic and pandemic risk transfer product availability and affordability,* including products for governments, corporates, individual households, and low-income populations.
- *Social protection policy,* recognizing that low-income populations should enjoy social protection, including social health protection or support in obtaining insurance coverage while insurance solutions for people that can afford the premiums should not be crowded out; and exploring the degree to which social protection complements or crowds out market-based solutions.
- *Unlicensed competition,* recognizing that the resilience of insurance providers depends on an adequate level of oversight. Unlicensed entities or those poorly supervised by agencies with insufficient insurance supervision and risk management expertise can destroy the image of insurance and leave their consumers without protection should a disaster cause their insolvency.

ADB provides details of the assessment tool.

The Public Sector's Coronavirus Disease Financing Landscape

2.1 Impact of the Coronavirus Disease Pandemic in Pakistan

18.   The COVID-19 pandemic in Pakistan hit a largely underfunded and under-resourced health system. Infrastructure, human resources, and health financing are low compared to surrounding countries (Figures 6a–6e).[7] The country's health spending per capita ($34) is the lowest among its neighbors, yet out-of-pocket payments are high at 54% (2020). The government's health provision system is weak, leading to 85% of total health expenditures (2016) being incurred in the private sector by patients across all wealth quintiles (Khalid et al. 2021).

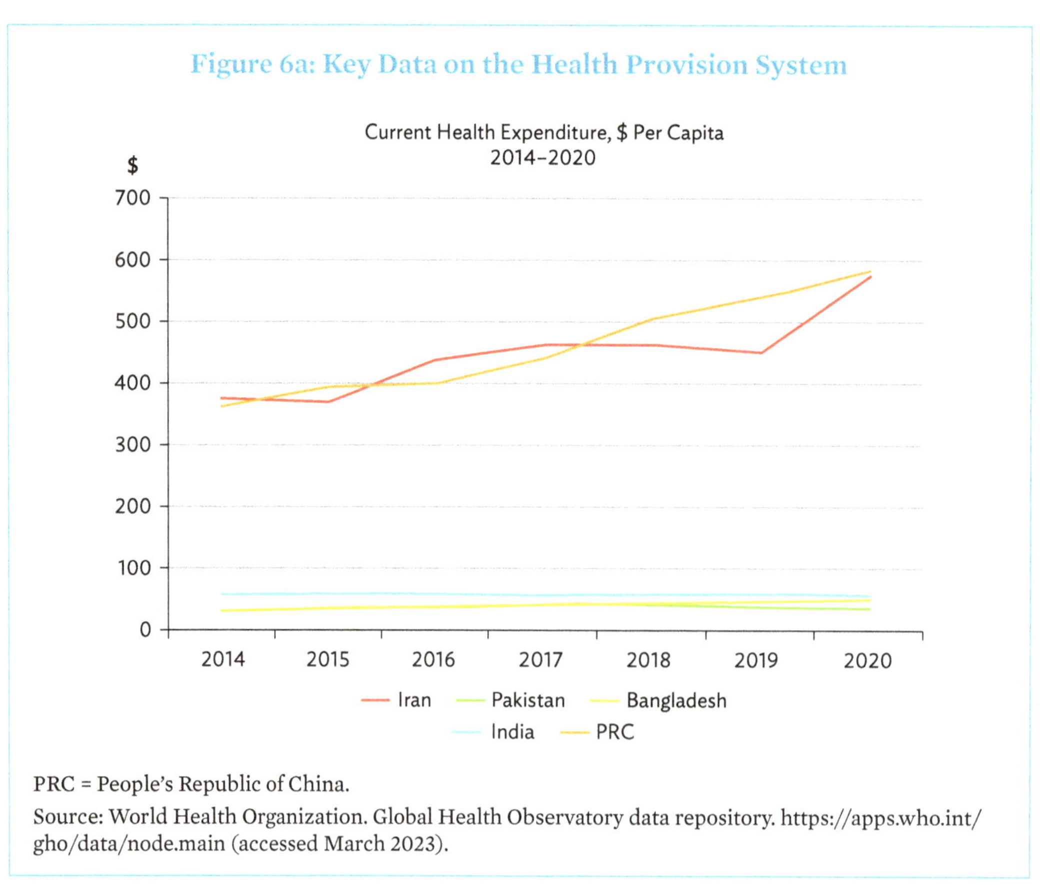

PRC = People's Republic of China.
Source: World Health Organization. Global Health Observatory data repository. https://apps.who.int/gho/data/node.main (accessed March 2023).

---

[7]   Source for all parameters in this para., if not otherwise indicated: WHO Global Health Observatory data repository. https://apps.who.int/gho/data/node.main.

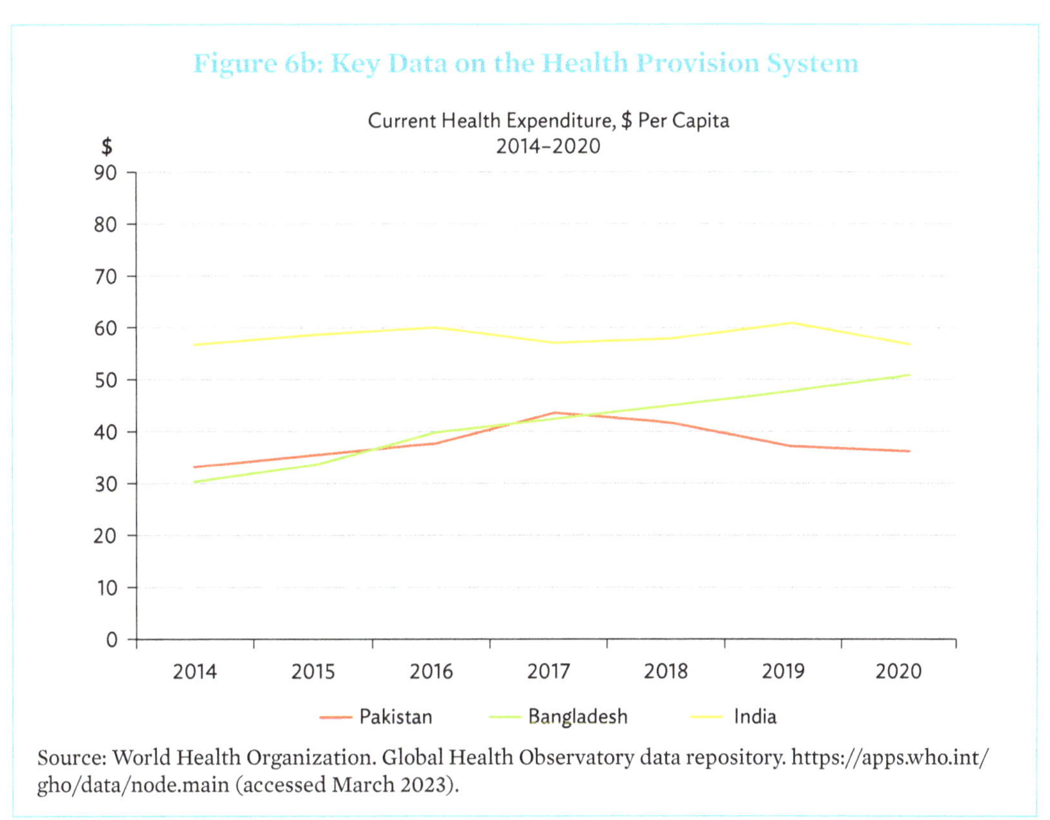

Source: World Health Organization. Global Health Observatory data repository. https://apps.who.int/gho/data/node.main (accessed March 2023).

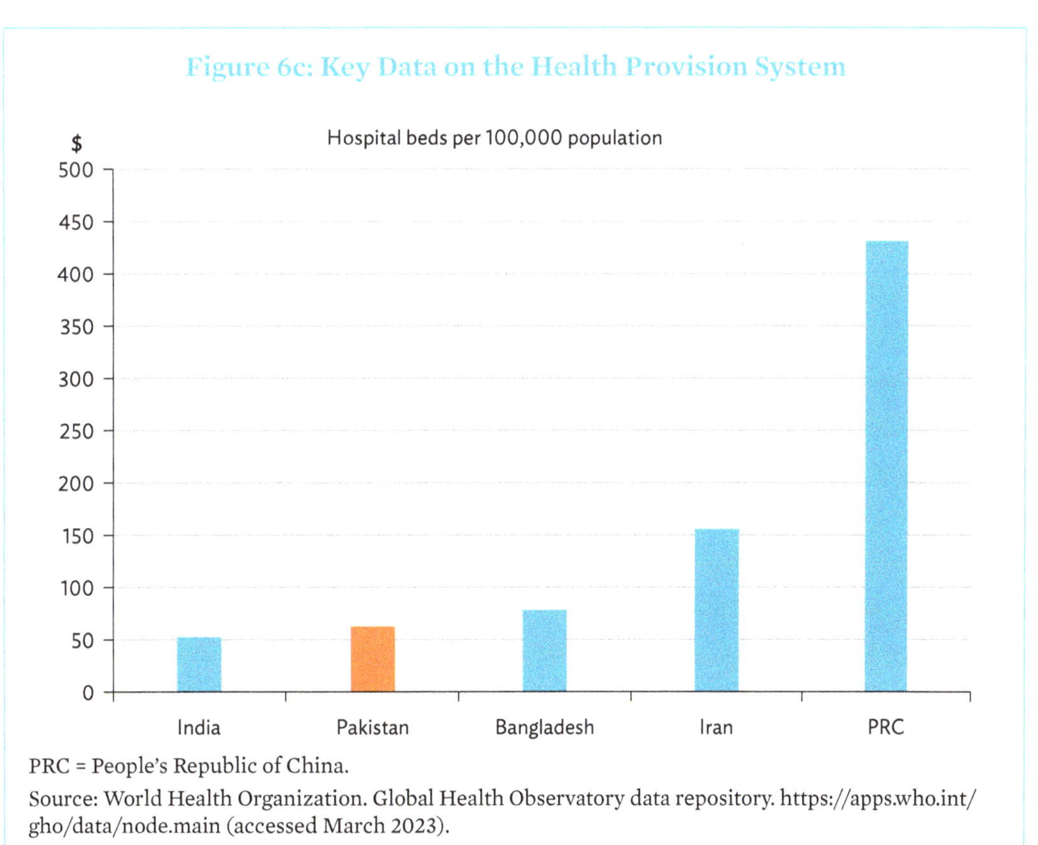

PRC = People's Republic of China.

Source: World Health Organization. Global Health Observatory data repository. https://apps.who.int/gho/data/node.main (accessed March 2023).

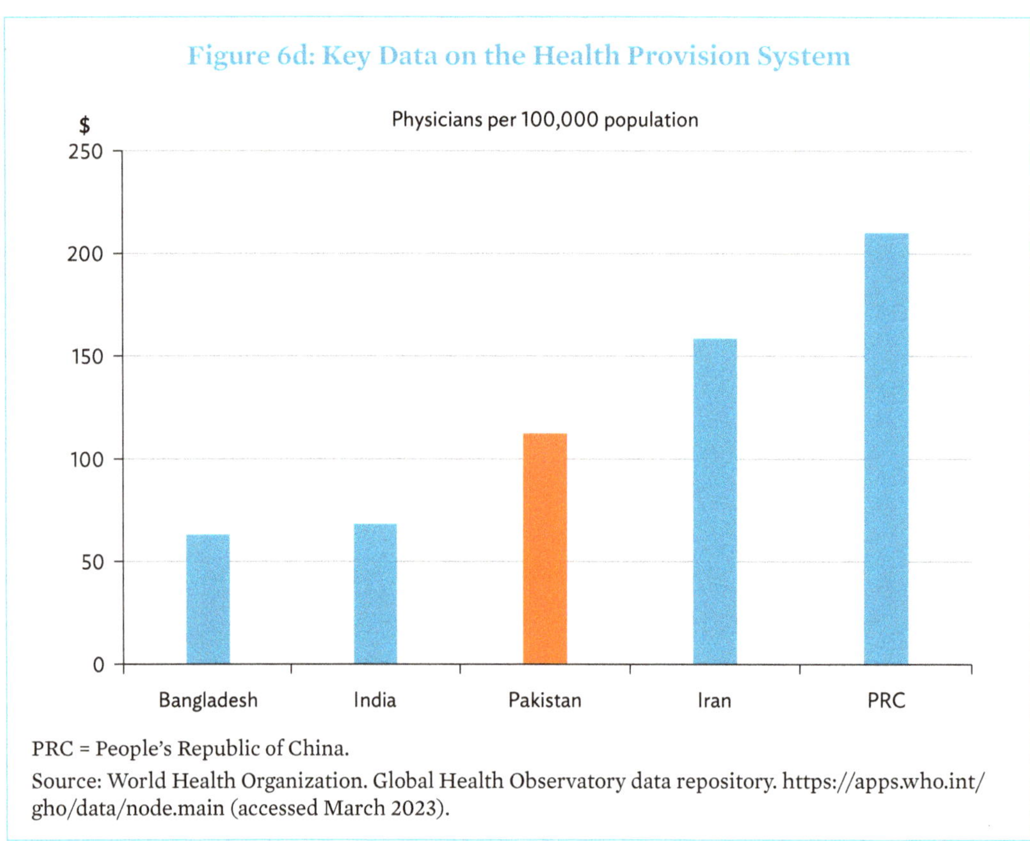

Figure 6d: Key Data on the Health Provision System

PRC = People's Republic of China.
Source: World Health Organization. Global Health Observatory data repository. https://apps.who.int/gho/data/node.main (accessed March 2023).

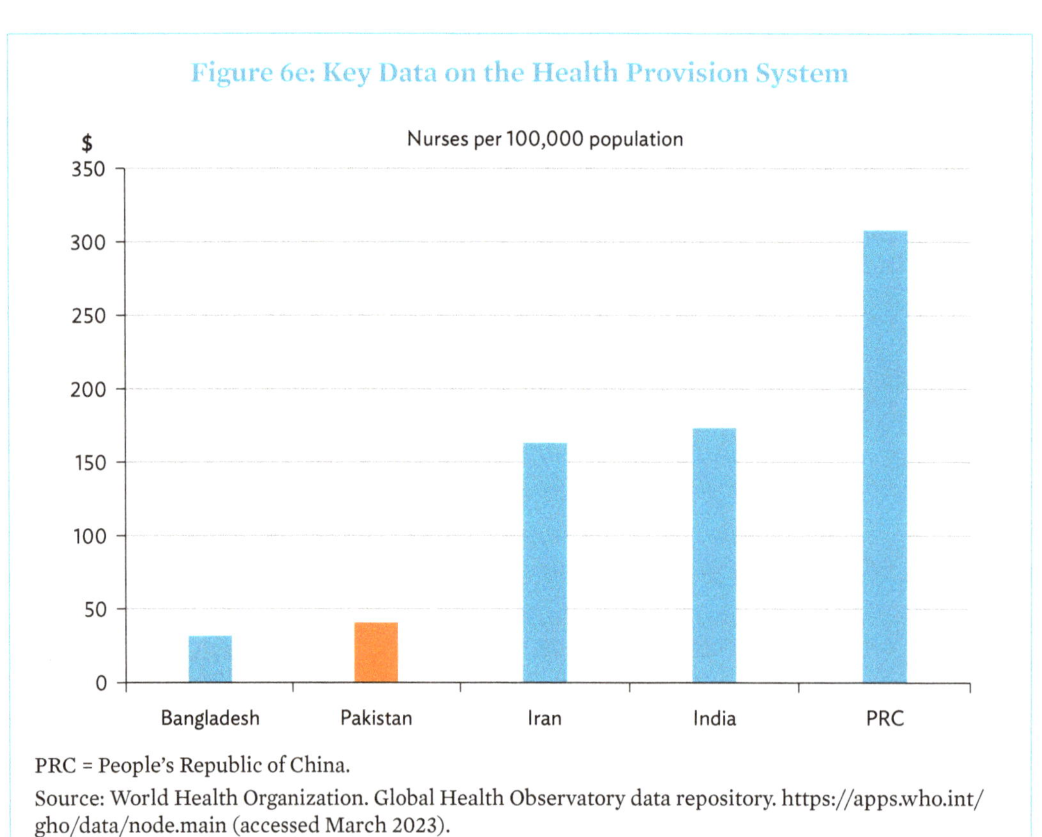

Figure 6e: Key Data on the Health Provision System

PRC = People's Republic of China.
Source: World Health Organization. Global Health Observatory data repository. https://apps.who.int/gho/data/node.main (accessed March 2023).

19.   The available health system infrastructure and resources were limited, especially hospital beds and nurses. The still comparatively high number of physicians may stem from the large share of practitioners in the largely unregulated private sector and its financial opportunities.

20.   The government took mitigating actions as the pandemic began, much as other parts of the world did. The first confirmed case of COVID-19 in Pakistan was reported on 28 February 2020. As the epidemiology and pathophysiology were unknown, even the clinical management guidelines were not clear to health care providers. Routine health care services utilization had dropped. Subsequently, the Ministry of National Health Services Regulations and Coordination developed standard operating procedures and guidelines on keeping essential health care services during the pandemic. Public hospitals (especially the secondary and tertiary levels) were designated for COVID-19 and non-COVID-19 services. If the need arose, the non-COVID-19 facilities would be added to the COVID-19 response. Due to the overall lack of resources, the government had to make available funding and commodities directly in an emergency reaction. Staff had to be redistributed to meet actual workforce needs. All COVID-19-related equipment were provided by the government to the designated hospitals, including oxygen supplies. Resource management software was developed to show the real-time data of services and resource utilization; however, this was not turned into a permanent system. Innovative measures were also taken. For example, Pakistan developed ventilators to an international standard when international markets ran out of supplies.

21.   As a precaution, the Government of Pakistan took several steps in responding to the pandemic. There were complete lockdowns, social distancing, and mask mandates, and surge capacity was built into public sector hospitals for the management of COVID-19 cases. The government established COVID-19 wards in all the public sector tertiary care and secondary care hospitals.

22.   Pakistan's reported COVID-19 caseload and its associated mortality was low relative to other countries, despite the backdrop of broader challenges in delivery of health services. As of March 2023, approximately 1.6 million cases were reported, with a total number of deaths of 30,643 (Figure 7). There were approximately 6,870 cases per 1 million population (compared to approximately 87,000 per 1 million population globally) and 13 deaths per 100,000 population (compared to 787 per 100,000 population globally).[8] These figures are clearly below the world average and can be explained with the fact that the COVID-19 pandemic was mainly focused on urban areas, while large parts of the population are living in rural areas with little contact to urban centers. For the same reporting period, 132,453,062 people were fully vaccinated (2 doses), while 139,714,655 were partially vaccinated in Pakistan. The national and subnational COVID-19 cases and associated mortality are given in Table 1.[9]

---

[8] Worldometer. https://www.worldometers.info/ (accessed 5 March 2023).
[9] National Command and Operations Center, Government of Pakistan. https://www.nih.org.pk/novel-coranavirus-2019-ncov.

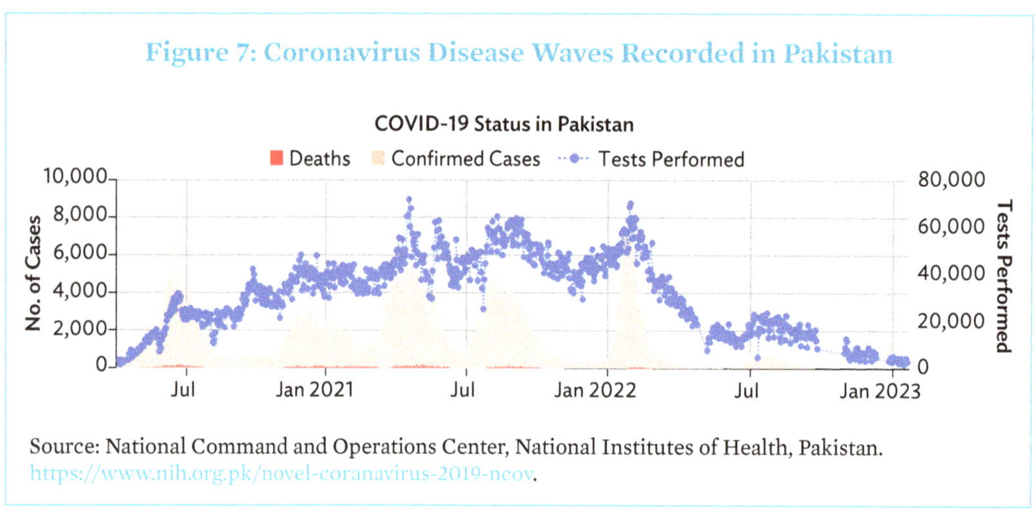

Figure 7: Coronavirus Disease Waves Recorded in Pakistan

Source: National Command and Operations Center, National Institutes of Health, Pakistan.
https://www.nih.org.pk/novel-coronavirus-2019-ncov.

Table 1: Coronavirus Disease Infections and Associated Mortality in Pakistan

Region	Confirmed Cases	Active Cases	Deaths	Recovery
Balochistan	36,068	582	378	35,108
Islamabad	140,283	5,112	1,031	134,140
KP	225,402	6,140	6,376	212,886
Punjab	525,376	19,967	13,623	491,786
Sindh	596,907	21,406	8,264	567,237
Other	56,595	1,548	984	54,063
Total	**1,580,631**	**54,755**	**30,656**	**1,495,220**

KP = Khyber Pakhtunkhwa.
Source: National Command and Operations Center, National Institutes of Health, Pakistan.

2.2 Institutions Involved in Combating the Pandemic

23.   Pakistan fought the COVID-19 pandemic with coordinated involvement from the whole government (Khalid et al. 2021 and Mirza 2021). The government had its entities working in close collaboration, including the Ministry of Finance, Ministry of National Health Services Regulations and Coordination, the Economic Coordination Committee, the National Command and Operation Centre (formed to combat the pandemic), the National Disaster Management Authority, and the provincial governments. The Prime Minister led the pandemic response through regular meetings with the Economic Coordination Committee. A government official noted that the Ministry of Finance made funds available for the medical response to the COVID-19 pandemic upon requests from provincial and national ministries and as per availability of resources. Budgets of other sectors and projects (e.g., education, delayed development projects in all sectors) had to be reduced, for instance in the health sector reallocating funding from slow-moving initiatives.

24.   The Ministry of National Health Services Regulations and Coordination had no contingency funding in place to respond to COVID-19 despite the 2017 WHO Joint External Evaluation's recommendation to set up a specific budget line and funding allocation for International Health Regulations/disease surveillance and emergency response. The ministry reallocated funding from slow-moving initiatives to support the COVID-19 response. The country also received significant international support of $860 million specifically for health-related COVID-19 response. The ministry budget reallocations impacted the delivery of other health services. The ministry indicated the need to establish discretionary funds in the future that it can access quickly for emergency purposes plus fast-tracked emergency budget approval processes. Its noted that Sindh Province has established a PRs1.0 billion emergency health fund and that the federal government should do likewise.

25.   Under the Constitutional Schema of Pakistan according to the 18th Amendment, the provision of health services is a provincial mandate. The Economic Coordination Committee, therefore, implemented the cabinet decisions through the provincial Chief Ministers. The existing structures and processes allowed for the swift transfer of available funds across national and provincial levels. The National Command and Operation Centre, headed by the Minister for Planning Development, was the key policy decision-making platform throughout the pandemic. The National Disaster Management Authority served as key implementation body. Following the COVID-19 experience, there are plans to establish a permanent National Emergency Operation Centre under the authority. The need for a stronger national disaster response was further underlined by the severe 2022 floods in Pakistan. That flood resulted in over 1,700 fatalities, displaced nearly 8 million people, and caused total damage and loss of $30.1 billion (Government of Pakistan 2022).

26.   The federal government had a lead role in defining the policy measures to respond to the pandemic. In consultation with the provinces, the federal government developed the clinical and administrative guidelines for containing the pandemic. The provincial machinery enacted the national guidelines on clinical and nonclinical interventions in letter and spirit.

27.   The National Command and Operation Centre served as the nerve center for articulating and unifying the national COVID-19 response. The center implemented the COVID-19-related decisions of the National Coordination Committee. The center was in-charge to collate, process, and analyze COVID-19-related data acquired through digital means and personnel knowledge from all parts of the country. Based on the data analytics, the National Command and Operation Centre provided recommendations to all the actors in the COVID-19 response, including the health and finance departments.[10] The National Command and Operation Centre kept the National Coordination Committee informed about the COVID-19 situation and response in real-time. Under the chairmanship of the Prime Minister, the committee would then set direction for the pandemic response. Box 2 presents key COVID-19 response interventions the National Command and Operation Centre led or supported.

---

[10] When the health system had needs, the Ministry of National Health Services, Regulation and Coordination would convey the same to the National Command and Operations Centre, and the National Disaster Management Authority, as part of the center, would make the provisions available to the health system. The National Command and Operations Centre also coordinated with the poverty alleviation division. For example, when the center recommended a complete lockdown, the poverty elevation division, under the Ehsaas program, distributed PRs134 billion to poor people.

Box 2: Coronavirus Disease Interventions Led by the National Command and Operation Centre

- Establishment of the COVID-19 National Helpline: 1166
- Establishment of a WhatsApp Chatbot for Health care Workers to register complaints.
- Launching and running of the Education Institutes Monitoring System.
- Supporting the Integrated Disease Information Management System.
- Launching of Pak Neghayban App for visualizing the availability of hospital beds and medical resources.
- Resource Management System for resource mapping of 4,000 COVID-19 and non-COVID-19 hospitals.
- Data-driven Smart Lockdowns in areas with higher COVID-19 positivity.
- Dedicated number of reporting standard operating procedures violations.
- Establishment of the Isolation Hospital & Infectious Treatment Centre.

COVID-19 = coronavirus disease.

Source: Authors.

28.　　　Sourcing material for infection prevention and control was challenging amid global supply chain disruptions. The National Disaster Management Authority took this challenge and did all procurements on the international market. Most of the materials were airlifted into Pakistan and distributed to the provinces through the provincial disaster management authorities. The national authority followed the procurement rules defined by the Pakistan Public Procurement Regulatory Authority. However, for emergencies like the COVID-19 pandemic, the National Disaster Management Authority law had exemption clauses to the Public Procurement Regulatory Authority rule, and the national authority exercised these exemptions for a rapid response to the pandemic. The Ministry of National Health Services Regulations and Coordination also invoked the exemption clauses in the procurement rules to expedite emergency-related procurements. These exemptions enabled direct negotiations with the suppliers and tax exemptions from the Federal Board of Revenue on importing goods. However, irregularities were reported, as discussed in the sections that follow.

2.3　Financial Support and Funding During the Coronavirus Disease Pandemic

29.　　　Funds were mobilized from both internal sources and development partners. International assistance was received in a combination of loans and grants (Table 2). The Ministry of Finance was the custodian of all funds. As indicated to the consulting team, whenever the National Command and Operation Centre and the National Disaster Management Authority required funds, they would send a request to the cabinet, and the Ministry of Finance would issue the requisite funds in full, within a week of cabinet approval whenever available. The COVID-19 funds were kept and managed separately. No other payments were made from these funds.

Table 2: COVID-19 Financing for Pakistan Preparedness Response Plan and National Vaccination and Deployment Plan: Health Component, December 2022

Donor/ Source	Grant/Loan	Window/Project	Purpose	Commitment in $ (million)	Funds Utilized Current Date $ (million)	% utilization
WB	Loan	Budgets of various existing WB projects across the country repurposed to COVID-19 activities Federal repurposed budget: **$8.50 million** Provincial repurposed budget: **$29.50 million**	Procurement of PPEs, Testing Kits, COVID-19 medicines through UNICEF	38.00	8.50 / 29.50	100 / 100
	Loan	WB new PREP financing restructured for COVID-19 vaccine procurement	Procurement of COVID-19 vaccine	158.00	155.00	**98**
	Grant	Pandemic Emergency Financing (in-kind support)	PPEs, testing kits, oxygen concentrators	15.00	15.00	100
ADB	Loan	Reappropriation of existing loans. Routed through NDRMF to NDMA for COVID-19 pandemic response.	For NDMA procurement of COVID-19 equipment	50.00	50.00	100
	Grant	Asia Pacific Disaster Response Fund. Government of Norway's Grant administered by ADB (in kind support)	Lab consumable and equipment	2.00	2.00	100
	Grant/In-kind	COVID-19 pandemic support; PPEs (in kind support)	PPEs and oxygen concentrators	3.00	3.00	100
	Grant	Support for capacity building of Disaster Management Institution - 4,500 HCW will be trained via HSA on management of COVID-19 patients in ICU	Capacity building of 4,500 HCW	1.72	1.72	100
	Loan	COVID-19: Vaccines procurement under APVAX facility	Procurement of COVID-19 vaccine	500.00	488.00	**98**

continued on next page

Table 2   *continued*

Donor/ Source	Grant/Loan	Window/Project	Purpose	Commitment in $ (million)	Funds Utilized Current Date $ (million)	% utilization
IsDB	Loan	COVID-19 Vaccine Procurement under IVAC facility	Procurement of COVID-19 vaccine	72.50	71.10	98
PRC	Grant/ Donation	Construction of Isolation Hospital and Infectious Diseases Treatment Centre (IHITC) in Islamabad	Isolation Hospital and Infectious Diseases Treatment Centre (IHITC) Islamabad	4.00	4.00	100
USAID	Grant	COVID-19: In-kind support via JSI: Strengthening of 154 DDSRU and 6 PDSRU	Strengthening of 154 DDSRU and 6 PDSRU	4.50	4.50	100
	Grant	TA Support via Chemonics: PoEs capacity building on surveillance management information system, online calculator and course for COVID-19 PPE, COVID-19 inventory management system developed	Technical assistance via Chemonics	2.50	2.50	100
	Grant	In-kind support via Chemonics: 200 ventilator delivered, installed, and relevant staff trained in various districts across the country	200 ventilators	4.00	4.00	100
Japan	Grant	Grant-in-aid	Equipment for tertiary care hospital	7.45	7.45	100
Subtotal				**862.67**	**846.27**	**98**

ADB = Asian Development Bank, APVAX = Asia Pacific Vaccine Access Facility, COVID-19 = coronavirus disease, DDSRU = District Disease Surveillance and Response Unit, HCW = health care workers, HSA = Health Service Academy, ICU = intensive care unit, IsDB = Islamic Development Bank, IVAC = International Vaccine Access Center, NDMA = National Disaster Management Authority, NDRMF = National Disaster and Risk Management Fund, PDSRU = Pakistan Disease Surveillance and Response Unit, PoEs = Point of Entries, PPE = personnel protective equipment, PRC = People's Republic of China, UNICEF = United Nations International Children's Emergency Fund, USAID = United States Agency for International Development, WB = World Bank.

Source: Ministry of National Health Services (Regulation and Coordination).

30.   To cope with the financial impact of COVID-19, on 24 March 2020, the Prime Minister approved an Economic Stimulus Package of PRs1.24 trillion. The package was divided into three components: (i) relief to citizens, (ii) support to business and economy, and (iii) emergency response (Figure 8).

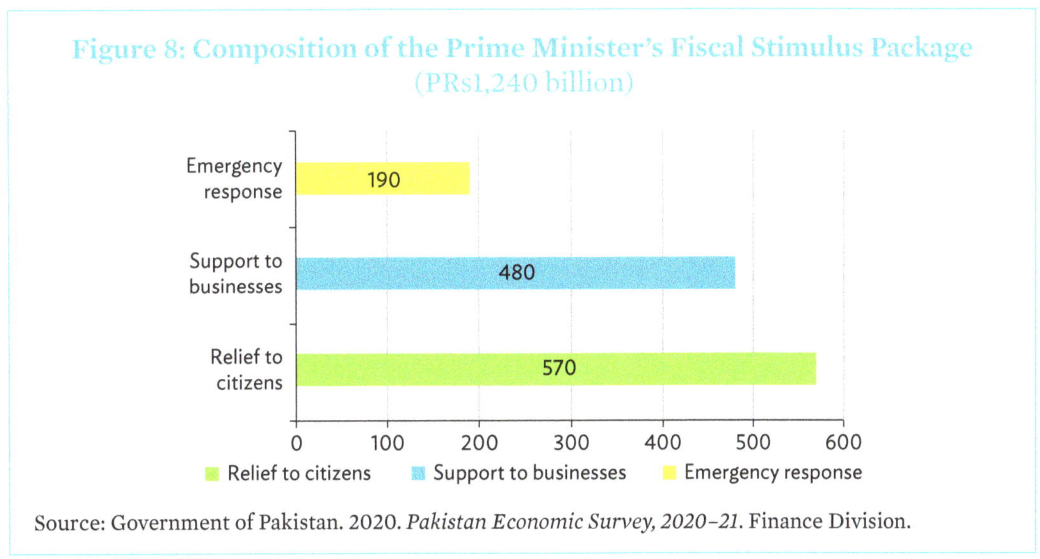

Figure 8: Composition of the Prime Minister's Fiscal Stimulus Package (PRs1,240 billion)

Source: Government of Pakistan. 2020. *Pakistan Economic Survey, 2020–21*. Finance Division.

31.   Most of the Economic Stimulus Package funds were allocated for relief to citizens (PRs570 billion) (Figure 9). PRs350 billion of this was allocated as cash assistance for daily wage workers and those living in shelter homes. A further PRs170 billion was subsidies on gas, power, petrol and diesel. PRs50 billion was allocated to the Utility Stores Corporation for provision of basic commodities (wheat flour, sugar, cooking oil, rice, and pulses) at a subsidized rate.

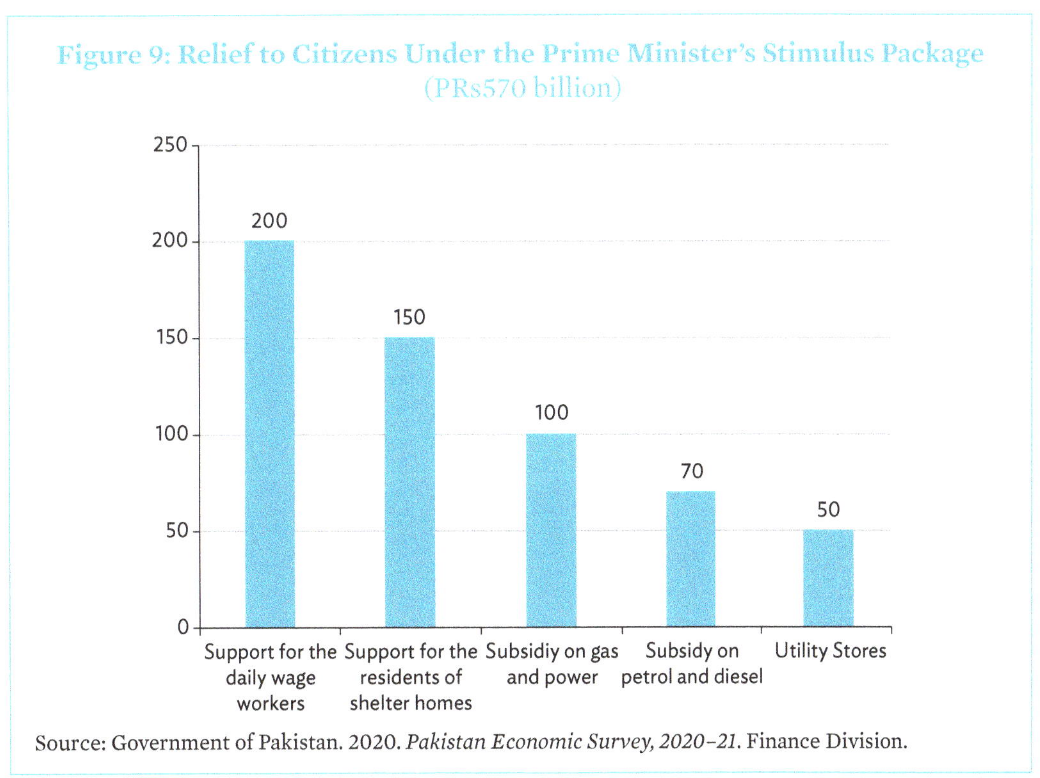

Figure 9: Relief to Citizens Under the Prime Minister's Stimulus Package (PRs570 billion)

Source: Government of Pakistan. 2020. *Pakistan Economic Survey, 2020–21*. Finance Division.

32.   A further PRs480 billion of the Economic Stimulus Package was allocated to support business and protect the economy. Figure 10 breaks down the components of the package.

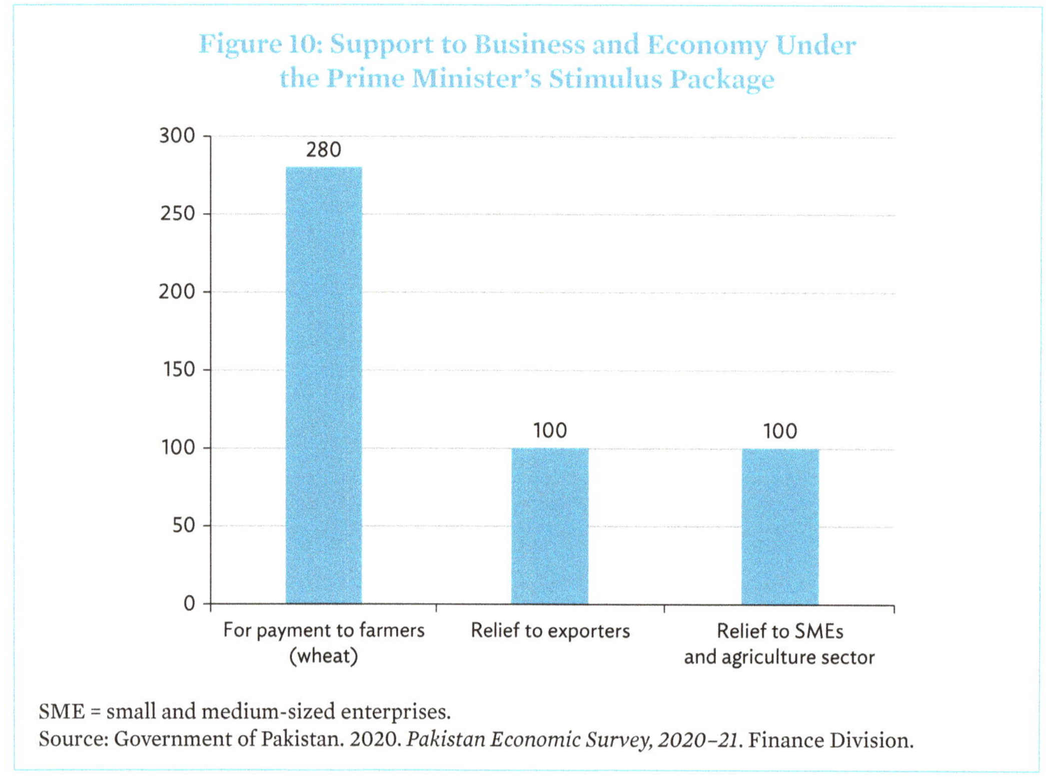

SME = small and medium-sized enterprises.
Source: Government of Pakistan. 2020. *Pakistan Economic Survey, 2020–21*. Finance Division.

33.   PRs190 billion of the Economic Stimulus Package was allocated for emergency (public health) response (Figure 11). Of this, PRs25 billion was allocated to the National Disaster Management Authority (for logistics, etc.), PRs50 billion for the purchase of medical equipment and incentives (allowances) for health workers, and PRs5 billion for tax relief on health and food items. PRs100 billion was kept as a residual emergency fund.

34.   In addition to the stimulus and relief package, the Ministry of Planning and Development allocated PRs70 billion for COVID-19-related expenditures in 2020. The main objective was to enhance hospitals' capacities, build COVID-19 specific isolation wards and increase the number of vital machineries such as ventilators and oxygen-providing equipment. Furthermore, the health sector obtained approvals of PRs10.5 billion under the Refinancing Facility offered by the State Bank of Pakistan. The government faced higher spending amid less revenue. In 2020, it spent more on vaccines, medical equipment, etc., and nonetheless targeted a budget deficit target of 7% of GDP. It was successfully managed, with a 7.1% at year-end. In the first few months of the pandemic (2020), the government had no allocation in the budget for COVID-19 response as the budget had been approved in June 2019. Then the Prime Minister approved the Economic Stimulus Package, and a supplementary grant of PRs350 billion was approved. A major amount went to the Ehsaas program. On the external side, the Government of Pakistan was supported through grants and loans from bilateral and multilateral partners, as explained under para. 29.

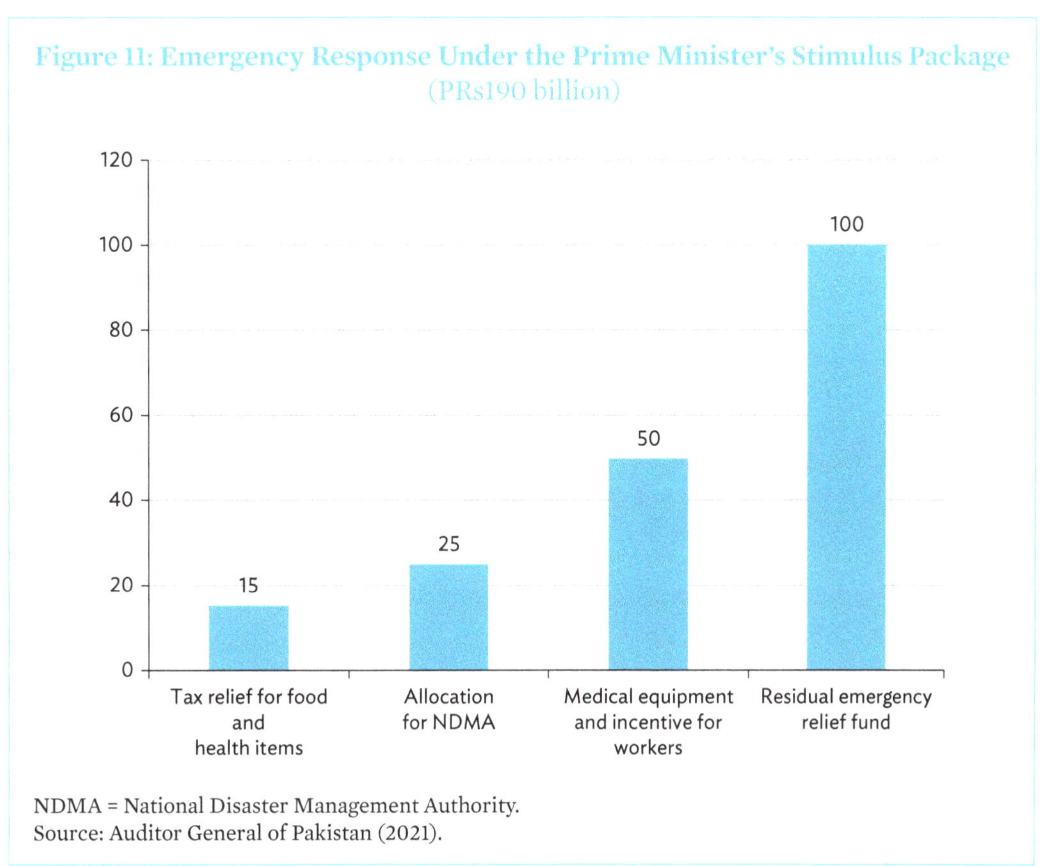

NDMA = National Disaster Management Authority.
Source: Auditor General of Pakistan (2021).

35.   Khyber Pakhtunkhwa officials noted that the federal government generously disbursed funds when needed by the provincial government for the COVID-19 medical/ infection control response at district levels. However, there were issues securing sufficient financing to support poor households throughout the pandemic.

36.   The Ministry of Finance, on receiving foreign exchange in grants and loans, provided support to the budget. The Ministry of Finance also provided a supplementary grant of PRs300 billion. Hence, PRs400 billion were allocated to the pandemic response in 2021–2022. Around PRs200 billion were spent by the seventh month of fiscal year 2021. Table 3 summarizes the total allocations for the COVID-19 response.

Table 3: Budget Allocation for Coronavirus Disease Response

No.	Description	Amount
1.	Prime Minister's stimulus package	PRs1.24 trillion
2.	Finance Department' supplementary grant	PRs40 billion
3.	Planning Departments PSDP allocations for health system strengthening	PRs70 billion
4.	State bank's refinancing facility	PRs10.5 billion

PSDP = Public Sector Development Program.
Source: Authors.

2.4 Diagnostic and Recommended Actions

37.   A federal coordination center for pandemic response (the National Command and Operation Centre) was established on an ad hoc basis. The COVID-19 response saw close coordination among government agencies federally and provincially. This was achieved through establishment of the center and strong government leadership. The 2016 WHO evaluation had recommended the establishment of such a body within the Ministry of National Health Services, Regulations and Coordination.

> *Put in place legislation, protocols, funding sources, etc., to facilitate the rapid mobilization of coordination centers in response to major disasters.*

38.   While the provincial governments are responsible for health, their insufficient contingent funds delayed the containment of the pandemic in some cases. The federal government took the leading role during the pandemic, activating federal contingent funds.

> *Review the current allocation of contingent funds for disasters, pandemics, and epidemics at the provincial level.*

39.   The Auditor General of Pakistan said that government departments lacked preparedness to respond to the pandemics and that weak financial controls were observed, for instance, advance payments without formal securities, payments of financial assistance to both spouses (against the policy of payment to one), and payments of cash assistance to those already insured under the Employees Old-Age Benefits Institute. Other areas flagged by the Auditor General report were procurements without need assessment, delayed delivery of purchased goods, and lack of warehousing facilities (Report of the Auditor General of Pakistan 2021).

> *Address any areas flagged by the Auditor General of Pakistan and provide guidance regarding exemption clauses to the Public Procurement Regulatory Authority rule.* This will allow timely procurement as needed to combat epidemics and pandemics at an earlier stage.

Assessment of Current Availability and Usage of Insurance, Reinsurance, and Capital Markets for Disaster Risk Financing

3.1 Economic Conditions and Other Support Functions

40.   Pakistan is a lower-middle-income country with a population of 207.8 million, as per the 2017 census. By 2030, its projected population will be 263 million. In fiscal year 2021, Pakistan had a tax-to-GDP ratio of 9.4%, with 62% of tax revenues derived from regressive, indirect taxes (Government of Pakistan 2020). The country spends around 3% of GDP on health care, of which 1.8% is private and 1.2% is public spending (Pakistan Bureau of Statistics 2018).

41.   Pakistan was highly vulnerable to the health and economic impact of COVID-19 (Ministry of Economy 2020). Of the total population, 56.6% had become socioeconomically vulnerable, and the International Labour Organization estimated that some 12.6–19.1 million people may lose jobs (Pakistan Economic Survey 2020–21). The GDP contracted in 2020 (Figure 12).

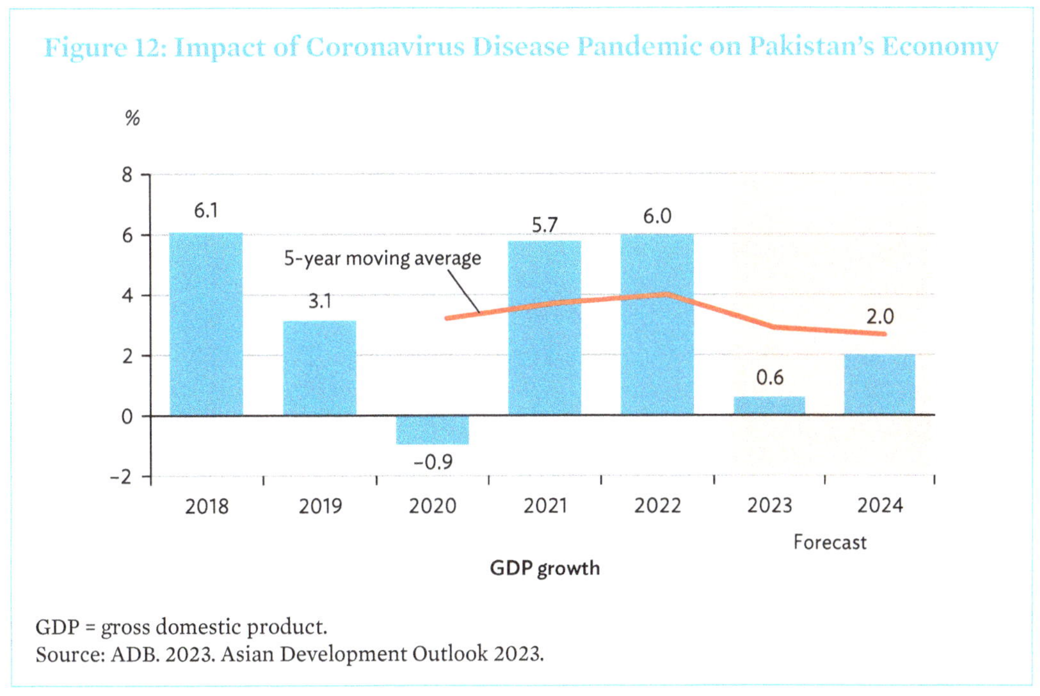

Figure 12: Impact of Coronavirus Disease Pandemic on Pakistan's Economy

GDP = gross domestic product.
Source: ADB. 2023. Asian Development Outlook 2023.

42.   The economic system's condition at the onset of COVID-19 was fragile. The multidimensional poverty head count stood at 38.3% in 2020. The contribution of deprivation in health to the Multidimensional Poverty Index was 27.6%. Given the socioeconomic vulnerability and weaknesses of the health system, the prospects of effectively combating COVID-19 were precarious.

43.   In 2016, Pakistan underwent a joint (Government of Pakistan and WHO) external evaluation for compliance with International Health Regulations and Global Health Security Agenda core capacities. The evaluation report highlighted that Pakistan lacked the capacity to (i) detect antimicrobial resistance, (ii) do surveillance of infections caused by antimicrobial-resistant pathogens, (iii) control and prevent health care-associated infections, and (iv) implement antimicrobial stewardship (WHO 2017).

44.   Based on those findings, Pakistan worked on various aspects of the 19 International Health Regulations core capacities. There were 4–5 key recommendations and then some area-specific recommendations. The Ministry of National Health Services Regulations and Coordination began pilot projects in three areas: the Integrated Disease Surveillance and Response, antimicrobial resistance, and pandemic control measures at the entry points. However, at the time of COVID-19 pandemic, these areas were not fully developed.

45.   In response to the joint external evaluation, Pakistan developed a national action plan for International Health Regulations core capacities. These plans were also costed. While the Ministry of National Health Services Regulations and Coordination was implementing the recommended actions, COVID-19 broke out. The systems were not fully prepared, but steps were already being taken in that direction. The Integrated Disease Surveillance and Response was still in a pilot phase in some provinces, and unable then to provide nationwide data.

46.   Despite progress during the pandemic, several deficiencies in Pakistan's pandemics preparedness were highlighted in the Global Health Security Index Report for 2021.

47.   The Global Health Security Index 2021 ranked Pakistan 130th among 195 countries. Pakistan's Index Score was 30.4 out of 100. The index ranks countries based on their preparedness to respond to global health security threats and assesses preparedness under six key areas: (i) prevention, (ii) detection, (iii) rapid response, (iv) health system capacity, (v) compliance with international norms, and (vi) risk environment (Bell and Nuzzo 2021). Pakistan scored 17.1 (compared to 28.4 global average) for prevention and 18.8 for response (against 37.6 global average). Pakistan's score for compliance with international norms was 45.8 (compared to 47.8 as the global average).[11]

48.   Pakistan scored "0" on eight of the 37 indicators: (i) biosafety, (ii) dual-use of research and responsible sciences, (iii) surveillance data accessibility and transparency, (iv) linking public health and security authorities, (v) medical countermeasures and personnel deployment, (vi) communications with health care workers during a public health emergency, (vii) infection control practices, and (viii) cross-border agreements on public and health emergency response (footnote 11).

49.   At the same time, Pakistan's options for complete or prolonged lockdowns were limited. The 2017–2018 Labor Force Survey showed that 61.7 million individuals were employed, with 23.8 million working in agriculture and 37.9 million in non-agriculture sectors. Informal workers made up 72% (27.3 million) of non-agriculture employment (Government of Pakistan 2020). Such a large chunk of informal employment limited Pakistan's options for complete or prolonged lockdowns. Nevertheless, almost 100% of micro-, small, and medium-sized enterprises were affected by the economic downturn and lockdowns, 30% had to shut

---

[11]   2021 Global Health Security Index (ghsindex.org).

down their businesses and more than 50% had to lay off workers and/or cut back salaries (Mohsin, Liu, and Ren 2020). Accordingly, the poverty rate has been estimated to have risen from 22% in 2018[12] up to 43% in April 2020, started to go down in May to 38.7% (IFPRI 2021), and recovered fast to 22% in September 2021 as stated by the government (Shezhad 2021).

50.   The health response to the COVID-19 pandemic was based on real-time data of the evolving situation, from the National Command and Operation Centre. The National Disaster Management Authority provided the capabilities and the platform for data management to set up a specific COVID-19 reporting system. This allowed Pakistan's Smart Lockdown strategy with geographically and temporally limited lockdowns.

3.1.1   Diagnostic and Recommended Actions

51.   The implementation of the key recommendations provided by the external evaluation for International Health Regulations and Global Health Security Agenda core capacities were interrupted by the COVID-19 outbreak. The focus of the government had to turn to combating the pandemics.

Continue to fully implement the key recommendations provided by the external evaluation for International Health Regulations and Global Health Security Agenda core capacities as reproduced below (and the results of the Joint External Evaluation in March 2023, forthcoming at the time of writing)

- Build the capacity to (i) detect antimicrobial resistance, (ii) do surveillance of infections caused by antimicrobial-resistant pathogens, (iii) control and prevent health care-associated infections, and (iv) implement antimicrobial stewardship (WHO 2017).
- Put the National Pandemic Preparedness Plan (2014) into action, finalize an all-hazard emergency preparedness plan, and mobilize resources to put these plans into action (WHO 2017).
- Map public health risks and resources to tackle the risks.
- Institutionalize the Disease Early Warning System and establish a regular mechanism to map resources and stockpile medicines and vaccines (footnote 12).

52.   At the onset of the COVID-19 pandemic, Pakistan suffered from a deficiency of human health resources, deficiencies in the routine health system data and limited availability of the public health laboratories. There were limited facilities for testing, tracing, and quarantine. The private sector did not contribute to the national data pool, and accreditation and governance for private providers were weak. The prices of diagnostic and therapeutic services in the private sector were not well regulated.

53.   The availability of insurance products covering both the health and business costs associated with pandemics and epidemics are largely affected by the risk reduction environment. For pandemics and epidemics, this is closely linked to a country's capability to manage communicable disease generally, and therefore, limit the risks of contagion.

---

[12] ADB. Pakistan and ADB: Poverty Data Pakistan. adb.org (accessed March 2023).

*Provide targeted investments in the health system to reduce epidemic and pandemic risk.
It is essential to make the health system more resilient by filling the human resources gaps,
especially of nurses and paramedics. A strong Integrated Disease Surveillance and Response
system and a network of public health laboratories across the country is needed.*

54.   Existing data systems are fragmented and not integrated and the data system for
COVID-19 case reporting had to be set up ad hoc during the pandemic. Further collaboration
with the private sector, better integration of the private sector in the country's health system
and governance, and enhancement of the digital health infrastructure according to the national
digital health strategy is needed. Pakistan is still struggling with the comorbidity data because
routine data is captured by vertical programs and hospitals, without integration. It needs to
structure the health data according to the International Classification of Diseases coding system.

*Work toward integrated and effective health data and reporting systems, integrating the
private providers.*

55.   The COVID-19 pandemic data has yet to be completed and used for the development
of epidemic and pandemic risk models. While real-time data on the evolution of the COVID-19
pandemic was made available, this data has not been used to develop pandemic and epidemic
actuarial models that could help the development of adequate risk transfer instruments.

*Use available COVID-19 data, once the National Disaster Management Authority has
completed collection, for the development of sophisticated pandemic and epidemic risk
models.* The models should be made available to government agencies, the insurance sector,
and other nonsovereign users, which may inform future pandemics and/or epidemics risk
protection product development.

3.2 Government Policy

3.2.1 Health System Structure and Regulation

56.   Pakistan has a pluralistic health system, broadly divided into civil (public and private)
and military (public) setups. The health system provides preventive, promotive, curative, and
rehabilitative services. However, the highest emphasis and finances go to the curative part,
i.e., hospital-based medical care. The National Health Accounts 2017–2018 has categorized
hospitals into three types: (i) public sector, (ii) private sector, and (iii) nongovernment
organization providers and/or nonprofit institutions (Pakistan Bureau of Statistics 2018).

57.   Due to the underfinanced network of public sector hospitals, people utilize private
health care more often. Availability, accessibility, and responsiveness play a vital role in the
public's choice to utilize the private sector. However, this has exposed people to significant out-
of-pocket expenditure on health care. The latest report of the National Health Accounts showed
that 56% of health care spending was out-of-pocket (Pakistan Bureau of Statistics 2018).

58.   Public sector hospitals work under the provincial health departments and are funded
by the respective finance departments. The finance departments largely plan their budgets
according to direct transfers from the federal government. Considering the low tax-to-GDP
ratio, the allocation for public sector hospitals has been historically low, pushing people

toward the private sector. Further, systematic underspending is a problem as institutions fail to execute their allocated budgets (Ghani 2018).

59.	Since 2015, the health care financing landscape has shifted significantly. In 2015, the provincial government of Khyber Pakhtunkhwa launched a social health protection initiative, called the Sehat Sahulat Program (SSP). In 2016, the Pakistan federal government launched the same program in Islamabad, Punjab, and other regions. These initiatives initially provided micro health insurance coverage to the population living under the national poverty line but have laterally expanded toward universal population coverage. The engagement of the insurance sector was part of the initiative.

60.	The 100% expansion to population entitlement under the SSP in Khyber Pakhtunkhwa started in 2021. More broadly, the federal government extended the 100% population entitlement from 2022 in a phased manner in participating provinces and regions. Apart from offering financial protection, these initiatives also successfully integrated private sector hospitals into the provision of public services at package rates agreed with the insurer.

61.	The SSP entitled 100% of Pakistani citizens to treatment within its packages. Beneficiaries' reach was limited due to challenges in accessing the services covered under the program. The challenges included lack of awareness and administrative issues (invalid and/or not updated according to the National Database & Registration Authority.

62.	Hence, claims have been equivalent to only around 50% of premium income, despite low premium rates charged to beneficiaries. The majority of unutilized premiums are handed to government (for Khyber Pakhtunkhwa, only reserves in excess of PRs2.5 billion are passed to the government). Federal and Punjab premiums are fixed for 3 years but for Khyber Pakhtunkhwa premiums are set annually.

63.	The SSP provided comprehensive inpatient cover, but disasters, pandemics, or epidemics were standard exclusions. However, Khyber Pakhtunkhwa supported COVID-19 treatment costs for 6 months (from February 2021 onward). Salient features of the SSP are given in Table 4.[13]

64.	There was a visible gap, as the Directorate General of Health Services and SSP responded with different approaches. People wanted to go to the private sector, but the directorate only responded through public sector hospitals, while SSP brought in the private sector. SSP Khyber Pakhtunkhwa identified 10 hospitals to provide services to COVID-19 patients, which were already on the program's panel and had service-level agreements with State Life Insurance of Corporation (SLIC). SLIC agreed on per-day service charges with these hospitals to treat COVID-19 patients. It paid the COVID-19-related medical claims from the SSP reserve fund.

65.	SLIC, on behalf of the government, managed the funds flow to private hospitals. Considering that the government of Khyber Pakhtunkhwa retained the risk, SLIC had no issue with the fund management. It was agreed that if the reserve fund is exhausted, the government will inject more money. An additional PRs4 billion was allocated to the reserve fund for the COVID-19 response.

---

[13] Social Health Protection Initiative Khyber Paktunkhwa. https://www.pmhealthprogram.gov.pk/.

**Table 4: Key Aspects of the Khyber Pakhtunkhwa
and Federal Sehat Sahulat Programs**

Description	SSP KP	SSP Federal
Region covered	Khyber Pakhtunkhwa	Islamabad, Punjab, Balochistan
Payer	Government of KP	Federal & provincial governments
Purchaser (insurer)	State Life Insurance Corporation	State Life Insurance Corporation
Providers (hospitals)	Both public and private hospitals	Both public and private hospitals
Eligibility	100% population (2021 onward)	100% population (2022 onward)
Entitlement	Secondary and tertiary care	Secondary and tertiary care

KP = Khyber Pakhtunkhwa, SSP= Sehat Sahulat Program.
Source: Khan, S.A. 2022. In-Depth Enquiry into the Implementation of a Large-Scale Social Health Protection
Scheme in the Context of the Drive Towards Universal Health Coverage in Khyber Pakhtunkhwa, Pakistan.

66.   COVID-19-related admissions remained a smaller part of overall utilization,
superseded by admission of dengue fever (epidemic) patients (Table 5).

**Table 5: Claims Under Sehat Sahulat Program in Khyber Pakhtunkhwa
for 2021, Comparing Coronavirus Disease and Dengue Fever
with Overall Admissions**

	Admissions		Expenditure (PRs)	
Experience	Number	Proportion	Mean	Median
Overall admissions	543,839	100%	24,976	15,000
Admissions for COVID-19	1,002	0.2%	375,536	225,000
Admissions for dengue fever	2,435	0.4%	7,368	5,600

COVID-19 = coronavirus disease, KP = Khyber Pakhtunkhwa, PRs = Pakistan rupees, SSP = Sehat Sahulat
Program.
Source: Sehat Sahulat Program Khyber Pakhtunkhwa annual report for 2021.

67.   Pakistan has both infectious and non communicable illnesses. However, as Figure 13
shows, utilization and/or spending under the SSPs (Khyber Pakhtunkhwa for instance)
remains largely on high-cost, non-communicable diseases.

3.2.2 Pandemics and Epidemics Risk Protection

68.   The legislative and executive authority relating to health care in Pakistan is vested in
the provincial governments. However, the Ministry of National Health Services Regulations
and Coordination has the primary mandate to meet national obligations under the global
health commitments.

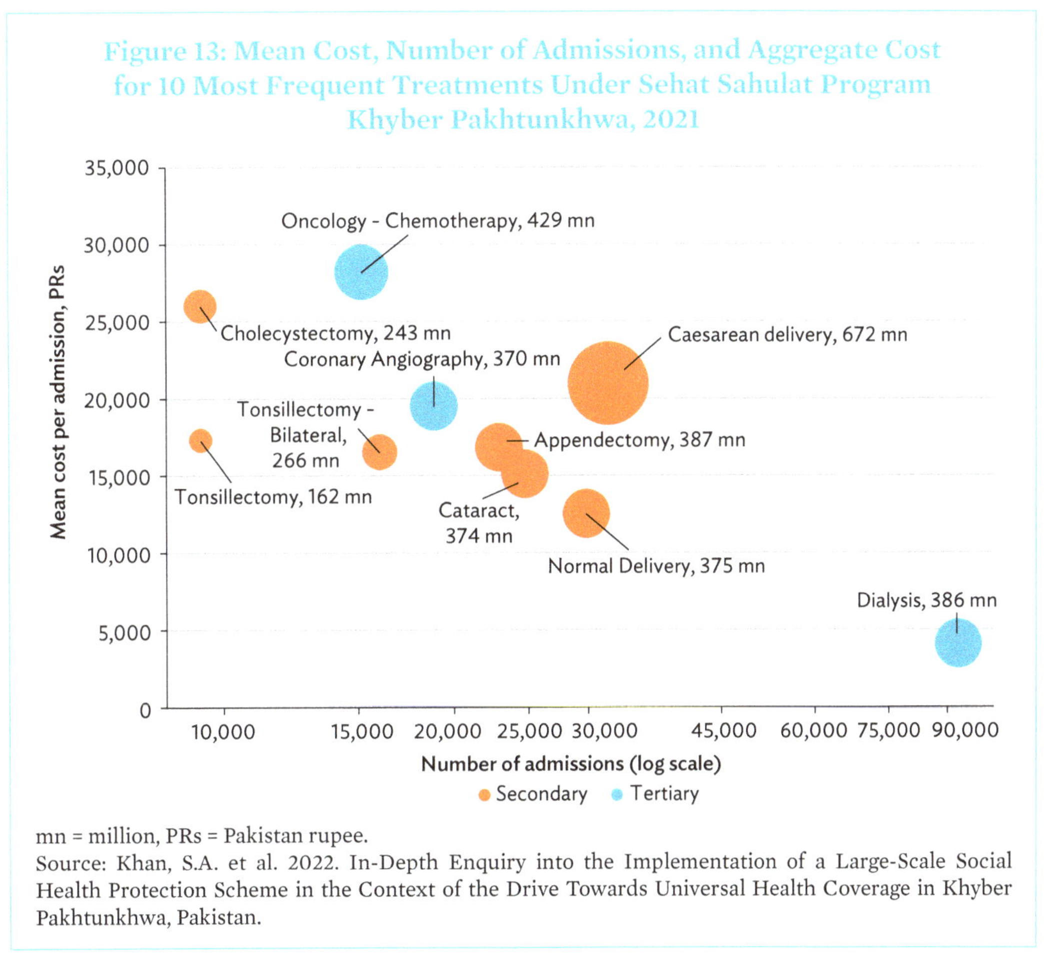

mn = million, PRs = Pakistan rupee.
Source: Khan, S.A. et al. 2022. In-Depth Enquiry into the Implementation of a Large-Scale Social Health Protection Scheme in the Context of the Drive Towards Universal Health Coverage in Khyber Pakhtunkhwa, Pakistan.

69.   The Ministry of National Health Services Regulations and Coordination, despite the transfer of power to the provinces, has the responsibility to deal with epidemics and pandemics. Due to the split in responsibilities, the federal government's role is less effective and limited to technical assistance and coordination of action plans between provinces.

70.   These arrangements worked previously in situations such as dengue outbreaks, but in view of the gravity of COVID-19, additional stakeholders entered the policy and implementation arena. These included the National Disaster Management Authority, the Provincial Disaster Management Authorities, and the National Command and Operation Centre (Box 3).

3.2.3 Financing of the Health-Related Expenditure on Coronavirus Disease

71.   Most funds for the health system's response to COVID-19 came from the federal government's stimulus package. The Ministry of Finance transferred the funds to the National Disaster Management Authority and the Ministry of National Health Services Regulations and Coordination. The federal government allocated:

72.   PRs70 billion ($456.6 million) for Integrated Disease Surveillance and Response and to strengthen the district-level hospitals on a cost-sharing basis with the provinces.

> ### Box 3: Federal Entities Involved in Combating Coronavirus Disease
>
> The National Disaster Management Authority, an integral part of the government's response to the COVID-19 pandemic, provided the logistics under the ambit of the National Command and Operation Centre. Provincial disaster management authorities, the provincial chapters of the authority, assisted the provincial governments in the pandemic response.
>
> The National Disaster Management Authority added 3,000 oxygenated beds to the health system and established a 250 COVID-19 bed isolation hospital in Islamabad with the support of the Government of the People's Republic of China. The authority also established and ran the hospital for 6 months and then handed it over to Ministry of National Health Services Regulations and Coordination. National Command and Operation Centre and the National Disaster Management Authority did not face major financial constraints while responding to the pandemic.
>
> The Ministry of Finance and Ministry of Economic Affairs were able to mobilize funds as needed by National Command and Operation Centre/National Disaster Management Authority.
>
> COVID-19 = coronavirus disease.
> Source: Authors.

73.   Around $900 million for the procurement of vaccines, in addition to over 124 million vaccine doses from the COVAX program.

74.   The government also received grants and loans from bilateral and multilateral development partners for COVID-19 response (Table 2).

3.2.4 Diagnostic and Recommended Actions

75.   Neither the Khyber Pakhtunkhwa government nor the federal SSP have funds allocated for responding to pandemics and/or epidemics. The reserve fund used to partly cover COVID-19 related-hospitalizations under SSP KP is a special fund, established to finance high-cost services like liver and kidney transplants and to purchase excess of loss coverage for the program but does not explicitly cover pandemics. Similarly, under the federal SSP, pandemics are excluded.

Implement a reserve fund for the federal SSP to help finance health care emergency, avert catastrophic health expenditure, and revise the benefits package to cover any pandemic or epidemic in the future. Future pandemic response should include all the SSP panel hospitals. Under the UHC Policy Board, Directorate General of Health Services and the Secretary of Health (in Khyber Pakhtunkhwa), as part of the policy board of SSP, should better fund SSP and Directorate General of Health Services pandemic response.

76.   Health care needs relating to the COVID-19 pandemic were financed completely by the government, with no risk transfer instruments supporting the budget. The financing of health system needs for the COVID-19 response were mainly borne by the federal government. SLIC (the sole insurer of SSPs) is a government-owned entity, and the inclusion of pandemic risks in the benefits package will have to be financed by the government. SLIC risk from SSP in part is retroceded to PakRe via a stop loss agreement (for federal SSP only). However, PakRe is smaller than SLIC and is government-owned as well. SLIC solvency is not linked to the SSP.

77.   The diversification of epidemic and pandemic risk is a central risk management challenge (The Geneva Association 2021). From a technical point of view, the insurance of

pandemics-related losses is problematic as geographic diversification of this risk, the central principle on which the benefit of insurance is based, is not possible. By definition of epidemics and pandemics, diversification of the risk within a country or globally, as for COVID-19, is not possible, making geographic diversification not applicable for the management of this risk. Capital market investors, too, are likely to steer clear of pandemic risk solutions, given the pandemic risk correlation with financial market impacts.

78.   Time diversification of epidemic and/or pandemic risk is possible due to the low frequency of severe epidemics and pandemics but the commercialization of such products is challenging. Diversification over time requires the design of multiyear policies. Such policies themselves present important obstacles in their commercialization: policies with a duration of more than a year are very seldom offered under general insurance due to volatility in frequency and severity and the commitment over years to pay for a premium is demanding.

79.   A complex payout design in line with the insurable interest principle is necessary. In addition to the multiyear duration of the policies, an effective insurance product for protecting the government budget will require a mechanism in the design of the product to match the financial demands generated by epidemics and pandemics. Thus, probably several payout triggers would be necessary to reflect their economic as well as health consequences and resulting public expenditure demands. Possible triggers could include bankruptcies, levels of unemployment, and hospital occupational rates. Designing such triggers that are objective, transparent, and not prone to fraud will need special expertise.

Explore possible acquisition of pandemic and epidemic risk transfer instruments that provide funds at the points of need for the federal government to enhance the risk-layered approach to epidemics or pandemics financing if economically viable.

80.   Given that health care needs relating to the COVID-19 pandemic were initially financed entirely by the government, a multipronged financial approach is necessary, using the various financing instruments together in the most cost-effective combination—and so applying a risk-layered approach. Utilization of development loan facilities, grants, and budget reallocations (important elements of the recent response), may not be the optimum way to finance future events as they postpone development projects or may result in the detriment of other sectors. To enhance pandemic and/or epidemic financing following the risk-layered approach, insurance and insurance-linked securities should be acquired if available at an economically viable cost (section 3.4.7).

3.3 Credibility of Private Sector Offering Risk Transfer Solutions

3.3.1 Insurance Regulation and Supervision of Health Insurance

81.   The pandemic exclusion on all insurance products except life offered in Pakistan limited the claims impact of COVID-19 to the sector. The Securities and Exchange Commission of Pakistan (SECP) did not come across any complaints regarding health coverage, nor on reinsured claims declined. Insurance sector investments, mainly held in government securities and corporate debts and bank deposits, did not see major shifts. Due to the pandemic exclusion in business interruption and travel insurance, no claims were made on these products. The on-site supervision was halted at the onset of the pandemic but a

few months later restarted with the use of digital platforms. A grace period for the statutory reporting and premium payments was granted, and digital sales platforms were allowed.

82.   The COVID-19 pandemic resulted in a significant reduction in new insurance business. The lockdown closed important sales channels like face-to-face sales and bancassurance, reducing new business by 50% in 2020 compared to 2019. Currency devaluation and inflation resulted in higher claims costs. On the other hand, the number of claims for several lines of business went down, especially for large motor insurance due to the diminished use of cars. Overall, the solvency of the insurance sector did not deteriorate.

83.   The main risk transfer instruments offered in health are the SSPs and/or universal health insurance products, however, those products are not approved by the SECP. They are governed under bilateral contracts between the government and the insurer. However, the Ministry of National Health Services Regulations and Coordination engaged the SECP to assess the proposal submitted by the insurance companies.

84.   SLIC is the current insurer, selected through competitive bidding by the Government of Pakistan (for the federal program) and the government of Khyber Pakhtunkhwa (for the KP SSP). These Social Health Program schemes are run by the insurer. The agreement with the insurer is of an administrative nature with limited risk transfer as the premium is yearly adjusted according to the claims experience. Pandemics are excluded in the programs and as such SLIC did not see the need for a premium adjustment due to COVID-19 with its loss ratio remaining at 65%–70%. The solvency and regulatory compliance by SLIC is supervised by SECP and no impact due to the Social Health Program's participation was reported. Neither SLIC nor private health insurance providers have international reinsurance in place.

3.3.2 Diagnostic and Recommended Actions

85.   A forward-looking supervision instrument in the form of stress testing of events like a long-lasting pandemic are not in place. The COVID-19 impact on the insurance sector was mild largely due to the pandemics exclusions in the insurance products. However, as the demand for pandemics protection increases and the economic effects of long-lasting lockdowns and economic downturns impact new production, surrenders, and fraud, the insurance sector's resilience will be tested. A forward-looking solvency assessment tool becomes necessary for effective supervision.

86.   Require the insurance sector to develop and carry out stress testing under epidemic and pandemic scenarios similar to the COVID-19 pandemic.

87.   The SSP benefits remain fully funded by the government and the participants, with no risk transfer to the insurance sector. The administrative nature of the agreement with the insurer to run the SSPs results in no risk transfer to the insurance sector. [14]

Consider transferring part of the health risk, including pandemic and epidemic risk, to participating insurers in the SSPs, with eventual support from reinsurance.

---

[14] The contract between SLIC and the government of Khyber Pakhtunkhwa includes an adjustment clause of the premium should the year end with a negative result for the insurer.

3.4 Product Availability and Affordability

3.4.1 Health Insurance Products

88.   Most of the health insurance products are corporate policies. There are very few individual health insurance products in Pakistan and the SSPs have further reduced the need for privately acquired health plans. The critical illness plans offered in the market do not include COVID-19 or other communicable diseases, like Ebola and Zika. This position of the insurance sector is unlikely to change in the short time given the challenges in managing these diseases through risk diversification techniques central to the insurance activity and thus the high required risk premiums that would jeopardize the demand for health insurance products (see para. 68–70 for a discussion of the challenges and possibilities to diversify pandemics and/or epidemics risk).

3.4.2 Diagnostic and Recommended Actions

89.   All health-claims-related data from the SSPs is only available to the government and SLIC, hindering an efficient pricing of supplementary health insurance products by the whole insurance sector. The SSPs have significantly reduced the need for health insurance products, especially for the low- and middle-income population. Notwithstanding the decline in demand for health insurance products (which was already small before the introduction of the government-financed SSP), the insurance sector sees business opportunities in the health sector to supplement the SSPs, for instance adding executive rooms (single occupancy), higher limits for medical conditions, a wider range of treatments, treatments outside the country and second opinion, etc.

90.   Make the large health utilization data from the SSPs available to the insurance sector while complying with privacy regulations. *This will promote efficient participation of the insurance sector to provide supplementary health insurance products at an actuarial fair price derived from adequate pandemic and epidemic modeling that need to be developed.*

3.4.3 Business Interruption Insurance

91.   Business interruption or loss of income insurance is offered in Pakistan, but uptake is limited and the cover excludes pandemics and epidemics. The standard product is always linked to fire or property insurance and payout under the business interruption policy requires physical damage of the property. Pandemic-related business interruption or loss of income is thus not covered. Public awareness of the benefits of business interruption is also low and underwriting business interruption or loss of income requires transparency in the income of the insured, which is a challenge in most developing countries.

92.   Significant pandemic-related business revenue losses have remained uninsured. The COVID-19 combat measures in the form of lockdowns, limits on the size of gatherings, travel restrictions, etc., have led to negative GDP growth in many countries globally. The Organisation for Economic Co-operation and Development's (OECD) estimates show approximately $1.7 trillion in revenue losses in OECD countries for each month of confinement (OECD 2021) (Figure 14). The economic downturn affected 53% of households all over Pakistan as indicated by a 2020 survey carried out by the Pakistan Bureau of

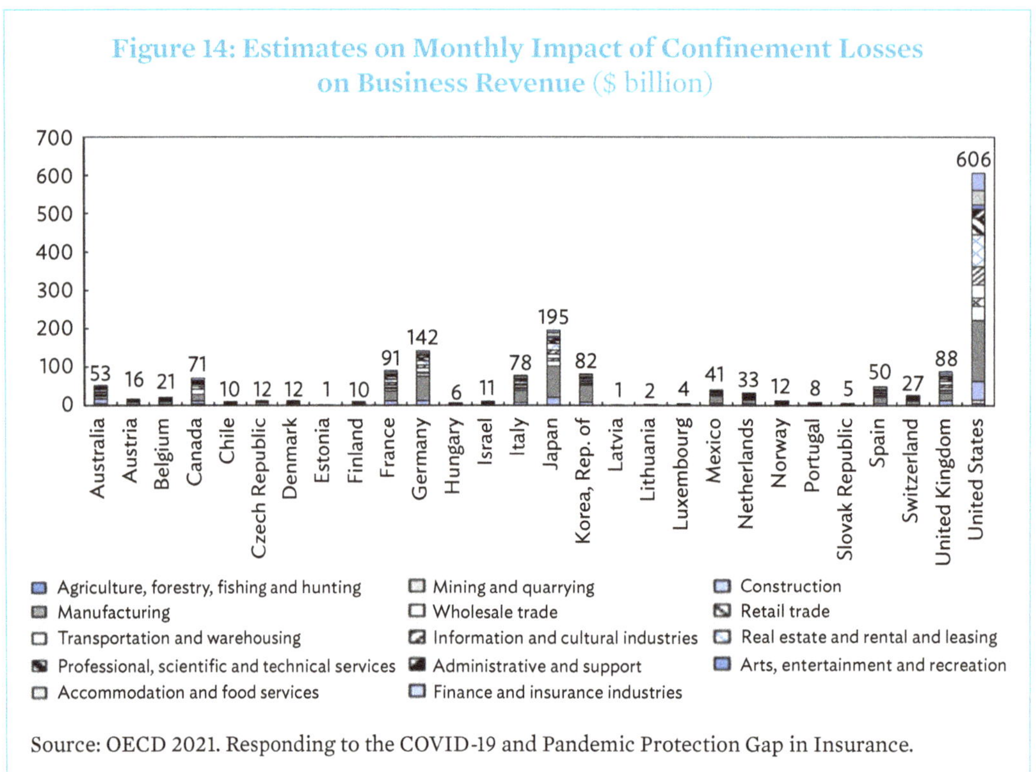

Figure 14: Estimates on Monthly Impact of Confinement Losses on Business Revenue ($ billion)

Source: OECD 2021. Responding to the COVID-19 and Pandemic Protection Gap in Insurance.

Statistics.[15] In Pakistan Economic Survey, 2021–22, 30% households reported that COVID-19 affected their psychological well-being substantially and 16% households reported more than 50% drop in their incomes.[16] In the absence of risk transfer instruments and to protect massive business closures and liquidations as well as exploding unemployment rates, governments globally have responded with significant financial support programs.

3.4.4 Diagnostic and Recommended Actions

93.   Lack of pandemic risk diversification and low demand for business interruption insurance need to be overcome for a viable risk transfer solution. Despite these difficulties, the private sector has offered such products for major events, such as the Wimbledon Tennis Championships. Such availability would benefit Pakistan.

Consider multiyear business interruption insurance that includes epidemics and pandemics from specialized insurers for the government budgets to allow for supporting businesses (paras. 91–92).

---

[15] Data also show that closure of businesses during lockdown from April–July 2020 had strong impact on the financial status of households. Some 53% of households all over Pakistan reported lower income, either earned or unearned; households in Khyber Pakhtunkhwa reported a 64% income reduction. The percentage is higher in urban areas as compared to rural areas with 67% and 63%, respectively. This may be because one of the main sources of income in Khyber Pakhtunkhwa is domestic or foreign remittances, which declined due to business closures (Pro Pakistani 2021).

[16] Finance Division, Government of Pakistan 2022. Pakistan Economic Survey, 2021–22.

3.4.5 Travel Insurance

94.   Standard travel insurance policies exclude epidemic and pandemic risk. One of the main reasons for this exclusion is that when an epidemic or pandemic is declared, it becomes a known event, contradicting the central principle of insurance that it should cover events that have not occurred or do not have a 100% probability of occurrence during the duration of the policy. However, during the COVID-19 pandemic, the requirement introduced for travelers in several countries to have a travel insurance policy that covers COVID-19-related costs led insurance companies to design such a product. This was possible due to the strict conditions for travel, such as full vaccination, negative testing, and quarantine.

3.4.6 Diagnostic and Recommended Actions

95.   Due to higher awareness of epidemic and pandemic risk, future travel insurance policies will have to include undeclared epidemics and pandemics in their coverage. This will only be possible at an affordable price if similar conditions that mitigate the risk are in place to travel, as was the case during the COVID-19, i.e., full vaccination, negative testing, etc.

Require future travel insurance policies to include undeclared epidemics and pandemics in their coverage.

3.4.7 Capital Markets Supporting Disaster Risk Transfer Instruments

96.   Issuance and trading of insurance-linked securities like pandemic bonds issued for the benefit of the government are not expected to happen in the near term. There has not been any issuance of less sophisticated insurance-linked securities such as catastrophe bonds in Pakistan so far, and the development of a pandemic or epidemic protection bond will require additional expertise. However, the further development of the capital market[17] will certainly create new financial instrument opportunities for the economy, including potentially for pandemics and epidemics.

3.5 Social Protection

97.   The long duration of the COVID-19 pandemic impacted the livelihoods of millions. In financial volume and needs, it revealed much higher risk financing for economic stabilization and social protection compared to direct health needs. According to a survey by the Pakistan Bureau of Statistics,[18] at the onset of the pandemic in 2020, around 20 million people lost employment (Figure 15).

---

[17] The Capital Market Development Plan and Vision 2025 of the government is supported by an ADB loan signed on March 2022. The intended ADB program will support the design and implementation of structural reforms necessary to create a competitive capital market and promote private investment in the country. https://www.adb.org/projects/documents/pak-53221–003-lna.

[18] Field enumeration of this survey was from 20 October 2020 to 5 November 2020. Results are prepared within 1 month of data collection or development and/or finalization of the questionnaire and methodology; various consultative meetings were held with relevant stakeholders, such as the Food and Agriculture Organization, World Bank, the United Nations Development Programme, the WHO, and the Ministry of Planning Development and Special Initiatives.

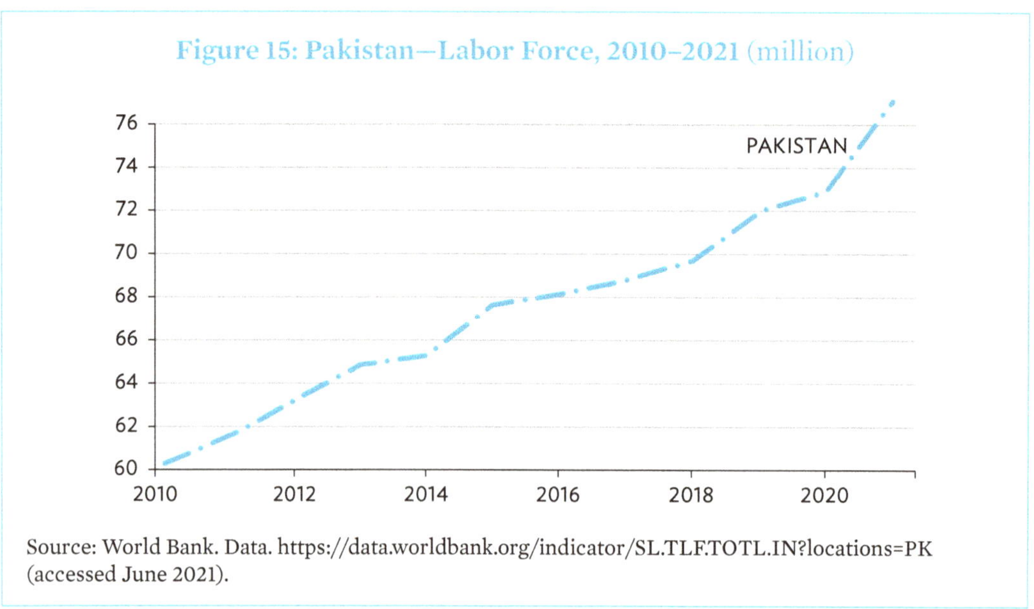

Source: World Bank. Data. https://data.worldbank.org/indicator/SL.TLF.TOTL.IN?locations=PK (accessed June 2021).

98.   The Ehsaas Program Pakistan actively supported people in distress during the COVID-19 pandemic. The Ehsaas Emergency Cash 2020 is an example of the protection of over 15 million daily wage earners and their households whose livelihoods had been reduced by the COVID-19 crisis.[19] However, and notwithstanding support from development partners,[20] the actual amount of the transfers (a one-off payment of PRs12,000 per family eligible), the duration of the support had to be reduced due to insufficient availability of funds.

99.   In line with the Ehsaas Program[21] 2021 poverty report,[22] a broader social registry and a denser network of payment stations will be necessary to cope with a future pandemic or epidemic of similar dimensions as COVID-19. The social protection response encountered two challenges in particular: rapid identification of the additional beneficiaries and/or those who fell into need of support, and outreach to the beneficiaries for the actual payments. With World Bank support, Ehsaas has recently updated the social registry and introduced digital access at local social protection offices.

100.   These challenges have led to further institutionalization of the Ehsaas programs. In response to the challenges, a single registration window for all Ehsaas social programs was launched on 8 June 2021,[23] and the number of Benazir Income Support Programme (BISP) beneficiaries has increased to 8.2 million according to the 2021 data (Ehsaas Program Pakistan 2023).

---

[19] For information, see the Ehsaas Program at https://ehsaasprogram.pk/.

[20] For instance, ADB's support to Pakistan's COVID-19 pandemic response in 2021 included a $500 million loan in August to help procure and deploy safe and effective vaccine, and a $603 million loan—of which $3 million is from the Asian Development Fund—for an integrated social protection program to strengthen Pakistan's flagship Ehsaas program. The loan is complemented by a $24 million grant from the Education Above All Foundation. See the ADB Member Fact Sheet at https://www.adb.org/sites/default/files/publication/27786/pak-2021.pdf.

[21] "Ehsaas is the most significant initiative of the Pakistan Government, especially the credit that goes to PM Imran Khan PTI. The primary aim of this program is to uplift the living standard of poor and needy people. In this Ehsaas program, 134 policies are working, and 34 agencies of the Federal Govt are given this task to implement it." See Ehsaas Program at https://ehsaasprogram.pk.

[22] See Ministry of Overseas Pakistanis and Human Resource Development (n.d.).

[23] The first prototype was opened in Sitara Market, Islamabad in July 2021. One Window Physical Centers of Ehsaas are planned in all 166 districts of Pakistan.

- ***Ease of registration in the Ehsaas programs.*** After online registration in the Ehsaas programs, each applicant is verified by the National Database and Registration Authority. The BISP then decides their eligibility and informs the applicant by SMS on their registered cell number. This number then grants automatic access to the different programs.
- ***Increment in the eligible person to the Ehsaas programs.*** The first BISP survey completed in 2011 had 23 variables to ascertain people in need but under its new name, Ehsaas Kafalat Programme, it has 43 variables covering a wider range of aspects related to the less privileged segments of society. As per the 2021 data based on the fresh survey, 3.4 million people have been added to the list of beneficiaries, resulting in 8.2 million BISP beneficiaries (Raza 2021). The National Socio-Economic Registry, which holds the data of the beneficiaries of the BISP, has been updated accordingly and can now be easily accessed through the single registration windows.

3.5.1 Diagnostic and Recommended Actions

101.   The importance of the Ehsaas is indisputable, but availability of funds was challenging due to the financial stress created by the COVID-19 pandemic and the competing needs for government funds.

102.   Acquire for the Ehsaas programs a risk transfer instrument that provides funds in the event of a pandemic or major epidemic, i.e., shock-responsive capacity, thus increasing its resilience when facing emergencies. *Such an instrument would support the funding of the Ehsaas programs when the effects of a pandemic or epidemic increase the number of eligible beneficiaries. It would also allow provision of additional benefits directly related with the pandemic and/or epidemic (see paras. 83–84 on the discussion of the availability and design of such risk transfer instruments).*

3.6 Unlicensed Competition

103.   Insurance activity is regulated and unlicensed entities or individuals providing or intermediating insurance would be acting outside the law. With the introduction of the Insurance Ordinance in 2000 "no person other than an eligible person or the branch of a body corporate incorporated in any jurisdiction outside Pakistan, which, immediately before the commencement of this Ordinance (Insurance Ordinance 2000), was registered to carry on and was carrying on such business in Pakistan, shall, after the expiry of one year from such commencement, continue such business."[24]

104.   The SECP controls unlicensed activity and its webpage maintains a list of companies engaged in unlicensed activity. The list, updated on 20 May 2022, does not contain any insurance unlicensed activity among the 93 companies engaged in unlicensed financial activities.[25]

3.6.1 Diagnostic and Recommended Actions

No recommendation is needed.

---

[24] https://www.secp.gov.pk/document/insurance-ordinance-2000/?wpdmdl=652&refresh=669fa67ab4b091721738874.
[25] The Social Health Protection Initiatives keep the hospitals operating at high occupancy so that they do not have room capacity to take on further patients that unlicensed insurance products, like prepaid programs, would bring in.

4

Conclusions

4.1 Rating Summary and Recommended Main Actions

105.   The ideal enabling environment for disaster risk financing (DRF) coincides with the achievable scenario for Pakistan. For this reason, the gap analysis of the current scenario has been carried out against the ideal scenario. Based on the insights gained by applying the W&W diagnostic tool, no differences between the ideal scenario and the realistic or achievable scenario were found. Responses from stakeholders regarding the realistic scenario were more by way of providing additional solutions for achieving the ideal scenario, rather than describing limitations that would hinder realization of the ideal. The figure presenting the ratings thus shows only the current situation versus the ideal enabling environment (Figure 16).

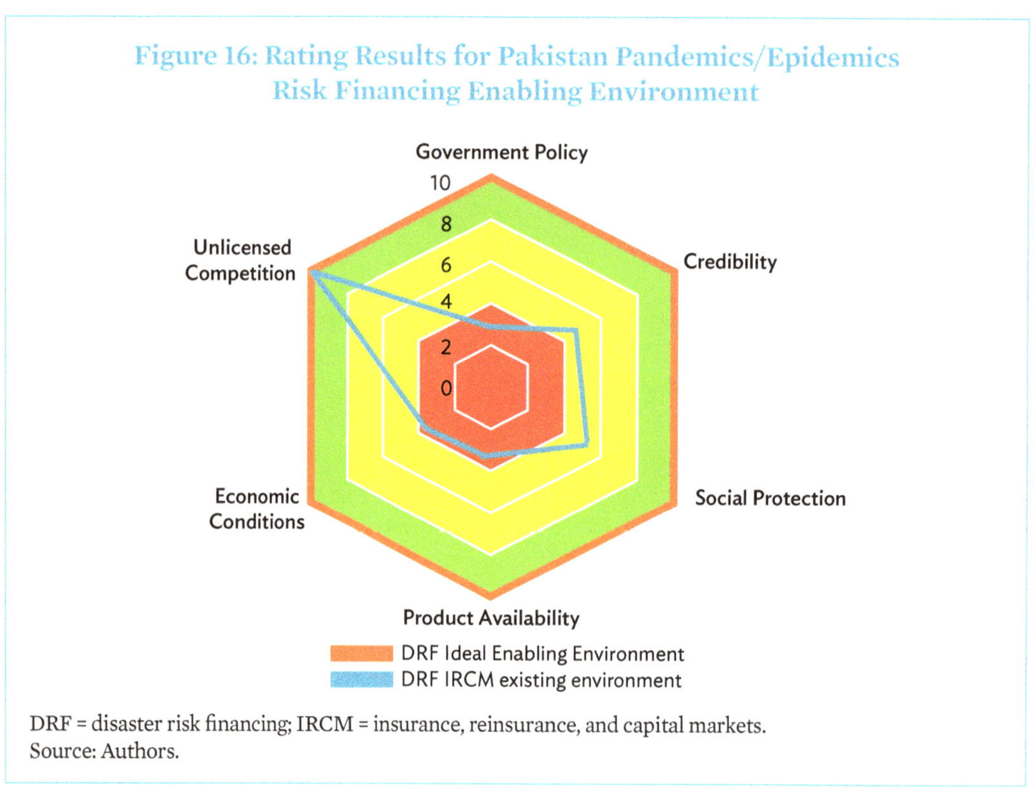

Figure 16: Rating Results for Pakistan Pandemics/Epidemics Risk Financing Enabling Environment

DRF = disaster risk financing; IRCM = insurance, reinsurance, and capital markets.
Source: Authors.

4.1.1   Economic Conditions and Other Support Functions

106.   The rating is in the yellow zone, implying need for action (sections 3.1 and 3.4.2).

Main gaps identified:

- The implementation of the key recommendations provided by the external evaluation for International Health Regulations and Global Health Security Agenda core capacities were interrupted by the COVID-19 outbreak.
- At the onset of the pandemic, Pakistan faced deficient human health resources, deficiencies in routine health system data, and limited availability of public health laboratories.
- Existing data systems are fragmented and not integrated and the data system for COVID-19 case reporting had to be set up ad hoc during the pandemic.
- The COVID-19 pandemic data has yet to be completed and used for the development of epidemic and pandemic risk models.

Main recommended actions to close the gaps:

- Continue the progress to fully implement the key recommendations provided by the external evaluation for International Health Regulations and Global Health Security Agenda core capacities.
- Provide targeted investments in the health system to reduce epidemic and pandemic risk.
- Work toward integrated and effective health data and reporting systems, integrating the private providers.
- Use available COVID-19 data, once the National Disaster Management Authority has completed collection, for the development of sophisticated pandemic and epidemic risk models.

4.1.2   Government Policy

107.   The rating is in the red/yellow border zone, implying an urgent need for action (sections 2.4 and 3.2).

Main gaps identified:

- A federal coordination center for pandemic response was established on an ad-hoc basis. The 2016 WHO evaluation had recommended the establishment of such a body within the Ministry of National Health Services, Regulations and Coordination.
- While the provincial governments are responsible for health care, their insufficient contingent funds delayed the containment of the pandemic.
- The Auditor General of Pakistan said that government departments lacked preparedness to respond to the pandemics and observed weak financial controls.
- Neither the Khyber Pakhtunkhwa nor the federal Sehat Sahulat Program (SSP) had funds allocated for responding to pandemics and/or epidemics.
- Health care needs relating to the COVID-19 pandemic were financed completely by the government, with no risk transfer instruments supporting the budget.

Main recommended actions to close the gaps:

- Put in place legislation, protocols, funding sources, etc. to facilitate the rapid mobilization of coordination centers in response to major disasters.
- Review current allocation of contingent funds for disasters, pandemics and/or epidemics at provincial level.
- Address any areas flagged by the Auditor General of Pakistan and provide guidance on the exemption clauses to the Public Procurement Regulatory Authority rule.
- Implement the federal SSP planned reserve fund to finance any unforeseen health care emergency or catastrophe and revise the benefits package to include pandemics and/or epidemics.
- Explore possible acquisition of pandemic and epidemic risk transfer instruments that provide funds at the points of need for the federal government to enhance the risk-layered approach to epidemics and/or pandemics financing if economically viable.

4.1.3   Credibility in the Insurance Sector and the Capital Markets

108.   The rating is in the yellow zone, implying a need for action (section 3.3).

Main gaps identified:

- Forward-looking financial supervision instruments in the form of stress testing of events such as long-lasting pandemics are not in place.
- The SSP benefits remain fully funded by the government and the participants, with no risk transfer to the insurance sector.

Main recommended actions to close the gaps:

- Require the insurance sector to develop and carry out stress testing under epidemics and pandemics scenarios like the COVID-19 pandemic (for the SSP).
- Consider transferring part of the health risk, including pandemic and epidemic, to additional insurers in the SSPs, with eventual support from reinsurance.

4.1.4   Product Availability and Affordability

109.   The rating is in the red/yellow border zone, implying an urgent need for action (section 3.4).

Main gaps identified:

- All health claims-related data from the SSPs is only available to the government and SLIC, hindering an efficient pricing of supplementary health insurance products by the whole insurance sector.
- Significant pandemic-related business revenue losses have remained uninsured.
- Travel insurance policies exclude pandemics.

Main recommended actions to close the gaps:

- Make all health claims-related data from the SSPs available to the insurance sector while complying with privacy regulations.
- Consider acquiring multiyear coverage for business interruption that includes epidemics and/or pandemics for the governments to support businesses.
- Require future travel insurance policies to include undeclared epidemics and/or pandemics in their coverage.

4.1.5 Social Protection Policy

110.   The rating is in the yellow zone, implying a need for action (section 3.5).

Main gaps identified:

- The importance of the Ehsaas is indisputable but availability of funds was challenging due to the financial stress created by the COVID-19 pandemic and the competing needs for government funds.

Main recommended actions to close the gaps:

- Acquire for the Ehsaas programs a risk transfer instrument that provides funds in the event of a pandemic or major epidemic, thus, increasing its resilience when facing emergencies.

4.1.6 Unlicensed Competition

111.   The rating is in the green zone, implying no action is needed (section 3.6).

References

Asian Development Bank (ADB). 2013. *Investing in Resilience: Ensuring a Disaster-Resistant Future.*

———. 2019. *The Enabling Environment for Disaster Risk Financing in Pakistan: Country Diagnostics Assessment.*

———. 2020. *Assessing the Enabling Environment for Disaster Risk Financing – A Country Diagnostics Toolkit.*

———. 2021. *Technical Assistance for Strengthening the Enabling Environment for Disaster Risk Financing (Phase 2).*

———. 2023. *Asian Development Outlook 2023.*

———. Forthcoming. Toolkit for Insurance, Reinsurance and Capital Market Solutions for Disaster Risk Financing (revised report).

ADB and World Bank. 2017. *Assessing Financial Protection Against Disasters: A Guidance Note on Conducting a Disaster Risk Finance Diagnostic.*

Auditor General of Pakistan. 2021. Audit Report on the Expenditure Incurred on COVID-19 by Federal Government.

Bell, J.A. and J.B. Nuzzo. 2021. Global Health Security (GHS) Index: Advancing Collective Action and Accountability Amid Global Crisis. https://www.ghsindex.org/wp-content/uploads/2021/12/2021_GHSindexFullReport_Final.pdf.

Bhutta, Z.A., F. Sultan, A. Ikram, A. Haider, A. Hafeez, and M. Islam. 2021. Balancing Science and Public Policy in Pakistan's COVID-19 Response. *Eastern Mediterranean Health Journal.* 27(8): pp. 798–805. https://doi.org/10.26719/emhj.21.016.

Ehsaas Program Pakistan. 2023. One Window Program 2023. https://ehsaasprogram.pk/ehsaas-one-window/.

Ghani, Asma. 2018. Less than Half of the Health Budget Used. *The Express Tribune.* 27 April. https://tribune.com.pk/story/1696195/1-less-half-health-budget-used.

Government of Pakistan. 2020. *Pakistan Economic Survey, 2020–21.* Finance Division.

Government of Pakistan. 2022. Pakistan Floods 2022: Post Disaster Needs Assessment. Ministry of Planning, Development & Special Initiatives.

International Food Policy Research Institute (IFPRI). 2021. Estimating the Economic Impacts of the First Wave of COVID-19 in Pakistan Using a SAM Multiplier Model. Discussion paper. https://www.ifpri.org/publication/estimating-economic-impacts-first-wave-covid-19-pakistan-using-sam-multiplier-model.

Khalid, F., W. Raza, D.R. Hotchkiss, and R.H. Soelaeman. 2021. Health Services Utilization and Out-Of-Pocket (OOP) Expenditures in Public and Private Facilities in Pakistan: An Empirical Analysis of the 2013–14 OOP Health Expenditure Survey. BMC Health Services Research. https://ecommons.aku.edu/cgi/viewcontent.cgi?article=1852&context=pakistan_fhs_mc_chs_chs.

Khan, S.A. 2022. In-Depth Enquiry into the Implementation of a Large-Scale Social Health Protection Scheme in the Context of the Drive Towards Universal Health Coverage in Khyber Pakhtunkhwa, Pakistan.

Khan, S.A., R. Shahab, and A.R. Khattak. 2022. First-Year Report on Services' Utilization under the Universal Population Coverage Conferred by the Social Health Protection Initiative (Sehat Card Plus) in Khyber Pakhtunkhwa, Pakistan.

Ministry of Economy, Government of Pakistan. 2020. Impact of COVID-19 on Pakistan's Economy: From the Perspective of International Financial Institutions. https://ead.gov.pk/SiteImage/Misc/files/EAD_Covid-19%20Impact%20on%20Pakistan's%20Economy%20(27_04_2020)(1).pdf.

Ministry of Overseas Pakistanis and Human Resource Development. n.d. Labor Welfare and Social Protection Expert Group. Recommendations to Implement on Mazdoor Ka Ehsaas. https://www.pass.gov.pk/Document/Downloads/MKEF.pdf.

Mirza, Z. 2021. Pakistan's Response to COVID—An Aerial View. *Think Global Health*. 8 July. https://www.thinkglobalhealth.org/article/pakistans-response-covid-aerial-view.

Mohsin, Shafi, Liu Junrong, Ren Wenju. 2020. Impact of COVID-19 Pandemic on Micro, Small, and Medium-Sized Enterprises Operating in Pakistan. Center for Trans-Himalaya Studies, Leshan Normal University. Leshan. https://www.sciencedirect.com/science/article/pii/S2590051X20300071.

Organisation for Economic Co-operation and Development (OECD). 2021. Responding to the COVID-19 and Pandemic Protection Gap in Insurance. 16 March. https://www.oecd-ilibrary.org/finance-and-investment/responding-to-the-covid-19-and-pandemic-protection-gap-in-insurance_35e74736-en.

Pakistan Bureau of Statistics, Government of Pakistan 2018. National Health. Accounts 2017–2018.

Poverty Alleviation and Social Safety Division. News release 2021. https://pass.gov.pk/userfiles1/files/Labour%20Day%20PR_May%201_Ehsaas_2021.pdf.

Pro Pakistani. 2021. Over 20 Million People Became Jobless in Pakistan Due to COVID-19. New release. 10 June. https://propakistani.pk/2021/06/10/over-20-million-people-became-jobless-in-pakistan-due-to-covid-19/.

Raza, Syed Irfan. 2021. 3.4 Million Added to List of Ehsaas Beneficiaries. *Dawn*. 23 August. https://www.dawn.com/news/1642078.

Shezhad, Rizwan. 2021. 22% of Pakistanis Living Below Poverty Line, NA Told. *The Express Tribune*. 28 September. https://tribune.com.pk/story/2322313/22-pakistanis-living-below-poverty-line-na-told.

The Geneva Association. 2021. *Public-Private Solutions to Pandemic Risk: Opportunities, Challenges and Trade-offs*.

Wehrhahn, R. 2010. Insurance Underutilization in Emerging Economies: Causes and Barriers. In C. Kempler, M. Flamée, C. Yang, and P. Windels (eds.). *The Global Perspectives on Insurance Today: A Look at National Interest versus Globalization.* Palgrave Macmillan.

World Health Organization (WHO). 2017. Joint External Evaluation of IHR Core Capacities of the Islamic Republic of Pakistan.

———. 2021. Global Expenditure on Health: Public Spending on the Rise? https://www.who.int/publications/i/item/9789240041219.

World Bank. 2020. Managing the Employment Impacts of the COVID-19 Crisis: Policy Options for Relief and Restructuring. *Jobs Working Paper.* Issue No. 49. https://openknowledge.worldbank.org/bitstream/handle/10986/34263/Managing-the-Employment-Impacts-of-the-COVID-19-Crisis-Policy-Options-for-Relief-and-Restructuring.pdf?sequence=4&isAllowed=y.

———. 2021. Updated Estimates of the Impact of COVID-19 on Global Poverty: Turning the Corner on the Pandemic in 2021? *World Bank Blogs.* 24 June. https://blogs.worldbank.org/opendata/updated-estimates-impact-covid-19-global-poverty-turning-corner-pandemic-2021.